JOYOUS
HEALTH

JOYOUS HEALTH

Eat and Live Well Without Dieting

JOY McCARTHY

PENGUIN

an imprint of Penguin Canada Books Inc.

Published by the Penguin Group

Penguin Canada Books Inc., 90 Eglinton Avenue East, Suite 700, Toronto, Ontario,
   Canada M4P 2Y3

Penguin Group (USA) Inc., 375 Hudson Street, New York, New York 10014, U.S.A.

Penguin Books Ltd, 80 Strand, London WC2R 0RL, England

Penguin Ireland, 25 St Stephen's Green, Dublin 2, Ireland (a division of Penguin Books Ltd)

Penguin Group (Australia), 707 Collins Street, Melbourne, Victoria 3008, Australia
   (a division of Pearson Australia Group Pty Ltd)

Penguin Books India Pvt Ltd, 11 Community Centre, Panchsheel Park,
   New Delhi – 110 017, India

Penguin Group (NZ), 67 Apollo Drive, Rosedale, Auckland 0632, New Zealand
   (a division of Pearson New Zealand Ltd)

Penguin Books (South Africa) (Pty) Ltd, 24 Sturdee Avenue, Rosebank,
   Johannesburg 2196, South Africa

Penguin Books Ltd, Registered Offices: 80 Strand, London WC2R 0RL, England

First published 2014

3 4 5 6 7 8 9 10

Copyright © Joy McCarthy, 2014

Design and food/prop styling by Carol Dano
Photography by Nicholas Collister

Manufactured in the U.S.A.

LIBRARY AND ARCHIVES CANADA CATALOGUING IN PUBLICATION

McCarthy, Joy (Nutritionist), author

Joyous health : eat and live well without dieting / Joy McCarthy.

Includes index.

ISBN 978-0-14-318691-5 (pbk.)

1. Cooking. 2. Health. 3. Diet therapy. 4. Cookbooks.   I. Title.

RM219.M34 2014   641.5′63   C2013-906535-0

Visit the Penguin Canada website at **www.penguin.ca**

Special and corporate bulk purchase rates available; please see
www.penguin.ca/corporatesales or call 1-800-810-3104, ext. 2477.

To my favorite lovebirds: my mom, Susan McCarthy,
and my dad, Michael McCarthy.

Mom—your sparkly eyes, passion for organic
gardening, baking talents and joyful spirit have
inspired me not only in the kitchen but in life.

Dad—your gentle soul and ability to look at the sunny side
of every single situation in life has given me the strength,
optimism and confidence to achieve my dreams.

. . .

CONTENTS

Introduction   viii

1   THE PATH TO
JOYOUS HEALTH   1

2   GET YOUR
GUT ON TRACK   19

3   FOODS, SUPPLEMENTS AND
HABITS FOR A JOYOUS MOOD   45

4   JOYOUS DETOX
SOLUTIONS   65

5   SUPERFOODS AND HEALTHY
LIFESTYLE HABITS FOR
JOYOUS HEALTH   85

6   CREATE A
JOYOUS KITCHEN   113

7   JOYOUS
RECIPES   133

Final Joyous Words   275
Food and Wellness Journal   276
Acknowledgments   279
Index   281

INTRODUCTION

In my early twenties I struggled with body-image issues, hormonal imbalance and digestive problems. For three years I visited countless doctors and specialists who performed every possible test you could imagine, searching for the "cure" for my hormonal imbalance—a cure I assumed would fix everything else. But after an exhausting three years, I was only getting worse. My skin was dry, my hair was thinning, I had not menstruated in over six months and I had *no* sex drive—ugh. I described myself as feeling like an "it." "Hopeless" was the perfect word to summarize everything I was feeling.

One night as I lay in bed with tears streaming down my face, trying to decide whether I should try yet another hormone-balancing pill to "fix" me, something inside was driving me to address the root cause. This yearning wasn't new, but this night it was stronger than it had ever been.

I said no to another medication and decided it was time for change.

Then it happened—some kind of magical and incredibly powerful paradigm shift occurred inside me. Whether it came from complete exasperation or a visit from my fairy godmother I'll never know, but I chose to take responsibility for my health.

Over the next six months I focused on healing my body from the inside out. I changed my diet, by adding, not deleting. I changed my thoughts, which turned into positive actions. And I followed the guidance of a holistic nutritionist and a naturopathic doctor—guidance I'm going to share with you in this book. It was a truly holistic approach.

Guess what happened? My hair began to grow back thicker and shinier, my skin was glowing again, and I actually got my period! I was jumping for joy. Slowly but surely all the symptoms I'd been struggling with for years became a fading memory.

I share this story with you to give you hope.

. . .

You always have the power of choice and the power to heal your body. You have choice over your thoughts, actions, words and every morsel you eat.

. . .

A few years later, I left my full-time marketing job and enrolled myself at the Institute of Holistic Nutrition, in Toronto, where I became a certified nutritionist and where I now teach. My certification enabled me to register with the International Organization of Nutritional Consultants and start practicing holistic nutrition, teaching others the healing power of food and healthy lifestyle habits.

Eat Well Feel Well was born in 2010, founded by Michelle Uy and myself as a six-week integrated holistic nutrition and yoga program in Toronto. I'm so proud of this program because it guides, empowers and inspires our students to learn a new way of eating *and* living without dieting or deprivation. This is the joyous health (aka ANTI-diet) way to live. In Eat Well Feel Well, you learn how to develop a new relationship with your body through yoga and, in doing so, with the food you eat.

I decided to write this book because I receive hundreds of emails, tweets and Facebook posts every month from people asking me for advice, or from out-of-towners who wish they could take the Eat Well Feel Well class or from those who found my Joyous Health blog and want to learn more but can't come and see me in person. I listened, and I have created this beautiful book for you so that no matter where you live in the world, you will have the information you need to heal your body and mind and experience joyous health.

This book comprises the entire holistic nutrition program that I teach in our Eat Well Feel Well class. It also has much more information to guide you and inspire you to eat well, and absolutely delicious (and nutritious) recipes that I am certain will inspire you and fill your belly with joy. And I have some very joyous news: You will notice as you work your way through my book that I never mention calorie counting. Free yourself from this forever!

Let the journey begin!

Joy

1
THE PATH TO
JOYOUS HEALTH

It's no wonder we are obsessed with diets when dozens of products with so-called health claims such as "low-fat" and "low-calorie" fill grocery store shelves. We are bombarded again while waiting in the checkout line by magazine covers promising the latest weight loss solution. And you can't turn on the television or listen to the radio without hearing about the latest diet fad or supplement that promises to melt fat off your belly, hips and thighs.

The madness stops here, with the truth.

There is no one-size-fits-all approach to health. What your friends thrive on or what melts pounds off the latest celebrity may be healthy and good for them but not necessarily for you. There are nearly seven billion people on this earth, and that means there are nearly seven billion ways to eat that can make each person thrive with joyous health. Diets are time-limited programs that promote deprivation. Basically, they make you feel guilty if you indulge in anything that isn't prescribed for that diet. Diets are not sustainable, period.

Getting Started

Ditch the "Diet" Mentality

A particular food can be one person's medicine while being another's poison. You are your own best nutritionist. But with that being said, you should consider taking a break from foods that you simply eat too much of too often. (We'll discuss these in chapter 4.) Keep in mind that it's not just about food. Lifestyle choices are equally important.

Stop Counting

Most people believe that counting calories and obsessing over a number on a scale will somehow make us reach an "ideal weight" and make us happier. But counting actually doesn't help, and in fact makes us feel worse about ourselves. Instead of focusing on a number, whether it's the number of calories, the number of fat grams or the number on your scale, focus on health and you will naturally choose the best foods for you.

Essentially, I want you to stop "nutritionalizing" your food. This means you should stop rationalizing your food choices with numbers. It's incredibly freeing when you realize you don't have to live your life from meal to meal, calorie to calorie. So instead of obsessing over numbers on nutrition labels, read the actual ingredients. Instead of obsessing over how much you weigh, focus on how you *feel*.

Eat Real Food

We live in a society that has, sadly, lost its connection with real, whole food. We've turned food into the enemy and become very disconnected from it by thinking of it as merely calories in and calories out. Let's fall in love with food again!

Choose foods that still resemble their original form. Michael Pollan shares a similar philosophy in *Food Rules: An Eater's Manual*—ask yourself, Was it picked from a tree, pulled from the ground, caught in the ocean? Many frozen dinners, fast foods and packaged foods hardly resemble what they originally looked like. I don't even consider many of these foods to be "real" food, but rather food-like substances. Choose more foods that don't even come in a package. Imagine choosing a food without a flashy health claim. The foods that don't claim to have health benefits are more often than not the most nutrient-dense—fresh fruits and vegetables don't come with food labels.

An easy way to reconnect with your food is to shop at a farmers' market, touch your food and prepare your own food. Strive to eat real food that is live, whole and beautiful as often as possible, but *find the foods that are best for you*. Don't worry, I will help you.

You ARE What You Eat, but Also What You Assimilate, Absorb and Don't Eliminate

Joyous health goes beyond what you put in your body. Healthy eating is nothing without good digestion, because poor digestion is the root of a great many illnesses. We'll learn more about this in chapter 2.

Listen to Your Body

Your inner wisdom will always guide you in the right direction. Trust yourself. You already have all the answers. Eat when you are actually hungry. Sleep when you are tired and rest when you need to. Push your body, because it is energized and rejuvenated by exercise, but don't overdo it. Let your intuition guide you to all the best relationships and have the courage to know when it is time to leave those relationships. Be kind to your body and choose thoughts that serve you well. We will talk about this more in chapters 3 and 4.

Be Proactive, Not Reactive: Think Prevention, Not Suppression (of Symptoms)

Every choice you make, every thought you think and every morsel you eat can move you closer to joyous health *or* closer to disease. You are ultimately responsible for your own health and well-being. You have the power to eat and think your way to vibrant health. You have choices! The key is to make these choices now, before your body is out of balance and you have to work twice as hard to get yourself back into balance.

Here is an example of how people become diseased.

Your body tells you, via symptoms of disease, when it falls out of balance. For example, you may keep getting colds or the flu; you may always feel tired, stressed or anxious; you may experience low energy, digestive problems or feelings of unhappiness. If you continue to ignore the signs and symptoms that your body is out of balance, you may become ill to the point that your doctor diagnoses you with a specific condition. He or she may then prescribe a pill to suppress those symptoms while never addressing the root cause of the problem. Further, some of these medications have significant side effects, and you may begin a vicious cycle of taking medications to counteract the side effects of other medications, all the while still not addressing the reason for the initial symptom.

The medicine that truly keeps you healthy right now is within the earth and within you—it's the food you eat, it's where you spend your time and it's how well you treat yourself and the company that you keep. You have all the answers within you to achieve vibrant joyous health.

Vibrant Health Is More Than Just Food

Joyous health is not just what you eat, it's also the way you live your life. Here are some important questions to consider on your journey to joyous health.

- How do you deal with stress?

- Do you make sleep a priority?

- What about your relationships—the people you surround yourself with and interact with daily? Are they emotionally healthy for you? Do you feel good after being with them?

- Do you get your heart rate up every day and move your body?

- How often do you connect to the earth (nature, fresh air, trees, grass)?

. . .

The words and thoughts you take in are just as important as the food you take in.

. . .

Your subconscious cannot distinguish between truth and fiction. It accepts your thoughts and words as reality. What an incredible opportunity you have! Your body will accept as the truth what you say and think on a daily basis. Do you fill your mind with loving thoughts, or do you have negative thoughts and say unkind things about yourself? Negative thoughts will promote stress, and stress will promote ill health and lower your self-esteem. You have choices! You are your own best cheerleader. You can have the life you desire and achieve all your dreams. You have the power to become the president of your dream company, if you so desire. Leaders don't succeed by telling themselves they aren't good enough, smart enough or attractive enough. Create the world you want to live in with the thoughts you keep.

Think Globally: Go Beyond Your Own Two Feet

When you think about how your choices will affect our planet, you will naturally make better choices. For example, try having a "Meatless Monday" every week. Why? Because the world's livestock accounts for 18 percent of greenhouse gases, more than all forms of transportation combined! Eating meatless just one day a week prevents more greenhouse gases than eating locally seven days a week. Why not do both? Go meatless on Monday and eat local, seasonal and organic as often as you can. Nurture nature and nature will nurture you.

What Is Joyous Health?

Joyous health is more than just the absence of disease or the avoidance of the occasional cold or flu. It is an optimal state of wellness not just physically but mentally and socially, characterized by:

- a positive mindset
- feeling *and* looking fabulous
- good digestion and elimination
- restorative sleep
- healthy relationships
- having energy for exercise and sex
- feeling joyous!

While it may not be realistic to expect joyous health 365 days a year, you should expect to feel well more days than not. You deserve to have joyous health, and I'm going to teach you exactly how to achieve it.

How This Book Works

I'm positively thrilled that you are about to embark on this wonderful and insightful journey to joyous health. Ideally it should take you six weeks to work through this book. However, you can take as long as you wish. Go at your own comfortable pace.

To get the most out of your journey, I encourage you to make time to read one chapter each week—this is your time to concentrate on you, because you deserve it.

I suggest you aim for one positive change per week, whether that is simply drinking more water (with lemon!) or practicing mindfulness when eating. This is a wonderful opportunity to steadily move toward a state of joyous health at your own pace. Just think, after a mere six weeks, you will have evolved in six different ways. That's amazing!

Set an Intention Each Week

An intention is a positive affirmation that will help guide you toward reaching your goals. It is something you plan to do, think or say to enhance your emotional, mental and/or physical well-being. Basically, it reminds you of your goals. Better yet, it is what gives you a little kick in the rear when you feel like giving up. Here are a few examples:

This week …
… I will drink water with lemon every morning to cleanse and detoxify my body.
… I will choose loving, positive thoughts about my body.
… I will choose healthy, delicious snacks that nourish my body.

Intentions empower you to take charge and enforce the discipline you have within you. Here's a quote I heard from successful businesswoman and entrepreneur Marie Forleo that I will never forget. The second I heard it, I wrote it down and taped it to my fridge: *Discipline is remembering what you want.*

It's really not surprising that research has shown you can use positive thoughts and self-affirmations to literally transform your life by bringing about behavioral changes. In fact, consciously reading your affirmation first thing in the morning can influence your decision making for the entire day.

Write down your intention and post it on your bathroom mirror or your computer monitor—somewhere you are going to read it every single day for the duration of the week.

Practice Mindful Eating

Does mindful eating mean you need to sit on a rock and meditate for 20 minutes before you eat your dinner? No, but that's not such a bad idea either! Mindful eating has been around for hundreds of years and has its roots in Buddhist teachings. Just as there are forms of meditation that include mindful breathing, standing, walking and sitting, mindful eating is an exercise to submerge your entire consciousness (and subconscious) in the act and enjoyment of eating.

You can probably relate to polishing off a bag of chips or a handful of chocolate chip cookies to numb yourself from frustrations at work or a fight with your significant other. When you practice mindful eating, you begin to free yourself from reactive negative patterns and instead eat because of *hunger* rather than for emotional reasons.

When you eat mindfully, you choose with deliberate intention to eat the foods that are the most nourishing and nutrient-dense. You will find that as you begin to make wiser food choices, you will also enjoy food *so* much more and realize there are more tastes than just sweet and salty.

Additionally, it takes approximately 20 minutes for your gut to signal to your brain that you are full. Too often, we eat too quickly—and end up eating too much because we're stuffed long before we know it. When you eat mindfully, you eat more slowly, and so you give this signaling a chance to occur.

Mindfulness in eating promotes balance and wisdom in all your food choices. Simply stated, it makes choosing healthy foods easier and prevents bingeing.

MINDFUL EATING HOW-TO

- Be involved in your hands-on food preparation as often as possible.

- Listen for and become aware of your physical hunger cues (warm feeling in your stomach) versus your emotional hunger cues (the desire to eat to numb or distract you from your feelings) to better guide you to know when to begin eating and to stop eating.

- Choose a peaceful environment to eat in without distraction—perhaps at your kitchen table with a candlelit place setting. Be sure to avoid eating in front of the computer or television.

- Once sitting, observe the food on your fork or place it in your hand. Notice its color and texture. Take a few moments to enjoy the beauty of this simple morsel before placing it in your mouth.

- Once you've placed this morsel in your mouth, actively use all your senses to joyously explore, smell, taste, feel and savor it. You have nearly ten thousand taste buds—use them to their full potential.

- Acknowledge your responses to food without judgment.

- Chew your food until it's almost a paste, and stop eating when you feel 80 percent satisfied (or when you know that after eight to ten more mouthfuls you would feel too full).

- Ponder the thought that you become the food you eat. Think about how the food you are eating will literally become the raw materials that build your body inside and out. Every morsel you eat will become waste or be utilized for one of any number of processes in your body, from thinking to creating energy at a cellular level or creating beautiful skin. Ask yourself whether you want to become a junk-food meal of a burger and fries or a beautiful, colorful, nourishing salad with a buttery avocado and garbanzo beans.

Choose one meal each day to practice eating mindfully.

Allow time for this meal, remembering that it takes 20 minutes for your stomach to signal to your brain that you are satisfied. You don't want to plan a mindful meal for when you are in a rush to be somewhere.

Breathe deeply, put your fork down between each bite and enjoy every morsel. With each bite, allow your taste buds and mouth to be fully engaged with all the flavors and textures. Close your eyes every few bites if that helps you focus.

Simple Habits for Joyous Health

Now that you've learned about setting an intention and eating mindfully, here are six new habits for joyous health. Choose one to focus on each week.

1. Take a break from coffee.

Most people want a stimulant in the morning—just look at the long lineups at coffee shops across North America before 9 A.M. However, when you've been sleeping for seven to eight hours, the last thing you should be putting in your body is a shot of caffeine. This provides only a short-lived burst of energy, because hormones that are released by caffeine stimulate the release of stored sugar into the bloodstream. This is not so great if you aren't using that extra sugar for energy and are instead sitting in your car or at your desk. If you're not active, excess sugar will eventually be converted to fat. This sugar spike will be followed by an energy crash—also known as the 3 P.M. slump—which may find you back at the coffee shop, this time craving cookies and chocolate.

Furthermore, coffee is a diuretic—it increases the rate of urination—and may deplete your body of water and essential minerals such as electrolytes, calcium, magnesium, potassium and sodium. The body is often dehydrated first thing in the morning, and what you should do is drink pure, clean filtered water to aid the body in flushing out toxins and improving energy production in the cells, instead of relying on "dirty energy" in the form of caffeine.

There is a time and place for caffeine. In fact, coffee can be good for you because it contains some antioxidants that are beneficial for heart health. Interestingly, a 2005 study done by the American Chemical Society concluded that most Americans get their antioxidants, including polyphenols and flavanols, from coffee. Then again, the average person is eating the standard North American diet of processed foods and sugars, a diet completely devoid of antioxidant-rich foods. So it is obvious why coffee would be their main source of antioxidants.

When else is caffeine acceptable? Drinking a shot of espresso before a workout, provided you are not already tired, may enhance athletic performance for some people. Coffee stimulates your adrenal glands to pump out the energy hormones epinephrine and norepinephrine.

However, most of my clients who run marathons have told me that sport gels with caffeine increase their need to have a bowel movement, which is not great when you are mid-race! This is because caffeine stimulates your digestive system to move waste products through at a much faster rate. That's why many people rely on coffee to have a bowel movement. Have you ever noticed that when you don't have your coffee, you don't have your morning BM? It's not a coincidence. This is when you need to address the root cause of your constipation. (More on that in chapter 2.)

Your gut needs adequate time to properly digest, absorb and assimilate nutrition from the food you eat. When you drink caffeine, your gut has *less* time to perform these functions. Sure, coffee may give you an energy boost, but it will be short-lived, because not only will you eventually come down from your high, but over the long term you may absorb fewer nutrients from your food because it's forced through your gut too quickly. This translates into less nutrition getting to your cells to be utilized as energy. This can become a vicious cycle.

Drinking coffee or caffeinated beverages such as espresso or an Americano once in a while is fine. Beverages containing caffeine such as sodas are a definite no-no! Also, be cautious with black teas. One or two cups are fine, but if you are drinking more than that, then black tea can be just as stimulating as coffee. If you are relying on it to start your day or get through the afternoon slump, then I have two solutions for you!

Joyous Tip

Need a java detox? If you drink coffee and it is your goal to cut back, it's important to do so slowly. Caffeine acts like a drug in the body, so when you suddenly remove the drug, your body will experience withdrawal symptoms such as "caffeine-induced" headaches.

Gradually cut out or reduce your coffee consumption to prevent withdrawal symptoms*. I recommend you follow this guideline.

Week 1: Cut back to one and a half cups of coffee a day.

Week 2: Cut back to one cup of coffee a day.

Week 3: Drink one Americano a day. (One shot of espresso contains only 75 mg of caffeine, while a mug of drip coffee can contain over 250 mg.)

Week 4: Cut out coffee completely and instead drink green tea, which has anywhere from 25 to 50 mg of caffeine per cup.

*If you are experiencing a headache, this is likely withdrawal symptoms; simply drink more water and give it time to pass.

HEALTHY COFFEE ALTERNATIVES

CHICORY

One of the best-known coffee alternatives is chicory root. It looks like coffee but has a more earthy taste. It's easy to find in most health food stores and spice shops.

How to enjoy it: Into a conventional percolator, French press or drip coffee cone, measure 2 to 3 tbsp (30 to 45 mL) dried chicory root for each cup (250 mL) of water. Jazz it up by adding some of the spices or sweeteners mentioned below.

TEECCINO

Teeccino is gaining popularity as a coffee alternative. It is a roasted combination of carob, barley, chicory, dates, figs, ramon seeds, almonds and dandelion root. It looks like coffee but smells and tastes spicy with a hint of sweet. It is even brewed the exact same way you would brew coffee. It is available in a range of flavors, including hazelnut, or you can add your own spices. Look for it in health food stores.

How to enjoy it: same as chicory.

Joyous Tip

Spice it up! Add a pinch of any of these to your coffee alternative before placing in a French press, coffee filter or cup: ground cinnamon, cardamom or cloves.
Sweeten it! Add a few drops of liquid stevia or some honey, maple syrup or coconut sugar.

Jennifer's Story

Jennifer was thirty-two years old, a successful lawyer with a high-stress job. She came to me for nutrition coaching because she wanted to lose 20 pounds and decrease her coffee consumption. She was drinking four to five cups of coffee every day, had sugar cravings every afternoon, and on nights when she had to work late, she was drinking coffee then as well plus munching on chips and crackers. I suggested she follow a coffee detox (see opposite page).

Three weeks later we had her follow-up session, and she was smiling ear to ear (not to mention she was positively glowing). She told me she had cut out coffee cold turkey the day after we met, and after a couple of days of headaches and feeling very sluggish she experienced absolutely incredible energy. Her skin was truly glowing because she was no longer dehydrated. She had also lost six pounds because, no longer craving sugar, she wasn't eating her typical store-bought muffin to go along with her afternoon coffee every day and had ditched the late-night munching.

2. Drink lemon and water.

Each and every morning when you wake up, and before you eat breakfast, squeeze the juice of a quarter or a half of a fresh lemon into 1⅔ to 2 cups (400 to 500 mL) of room-temperature or warm (not hot) filtered water. You want the water to be cloudy—that's how you know you've got enough lemon juice. If you are concerned about your tooth enamel, drink it through a straw (preferably a glass one). You can replace the lemon juice with a capful or two of apple cider vinegar, if you wish.

This simple habit truly sets the stage for the day and has incredible benefits:

It CLEANSES the body: Lemon water cleanses and detoxifies the liver by increasing the liver's detoxifying enzymes. Your liver is absolutely essential to your health and well-being. It has more than five hundred functions, many of them involved with detoxification.

It increases BILE: Sounds gross, I know, but lemon water stimulates the liver's secretion of bile. Bile, along with fiber, is a carrier of toxins. So when you have a bowel movement stimulated by drinking lemon and water, you are more likely to eliminate waste products.

It ALKALINIZES the body: Experts say that an acidic body is essentially a magnet for disease, and cancer cells thrive in an acidic environment. Lemon juice aids in making the body more alkaline—the opposite of acidic. (Although lemon contains citric acid, it does not create acidity in the body.) Lemon enhances your digestive secretions so that acidic wastes are eliminated more effectively. Food as medicine!

It helps prevent CONSTIPATION: This simple habit "gets things going" in the gut. Rather than the forceful nature of caffeine stimulating your gut to quickly push nutrients through, lemon supports the body's digestive system. In fact, you may find your bowel movements improve once you introduce this one habit to your day.

It gets you GLOWING: After a few weeks of lemon and water, you may notice your skin is brighter, and if you suffer from skin blemishes, you may notice a remarkable improvement. The health of your digestive system and your liver is directly related to the health of your skin.

It reduces HEARTBURN: I realize this sounds counterintuitive, but the majority of people with heartburn are actually under-producing stomach acid. When you strengthen your digestive secretions with lemon and water, you may notice an incredible improvement in your heartburn.

You will be amazed at how good you feel after drinking lemon with water for just one week. I have been advising my clients to do this for years, and I'm not the only nutrition expert who recommends this daily ritual for health, well-being and detoxification. In fact, people around the world have been doing this for hundreds of years!

3. Think veggie-centric.

At every meal and snack, make sure your plate contains some vegetables. These mighty powerful foods are a rich source of nutrients, including vitamins A, B-complex, C and K, protein, minerals, antioxidants and fiber. Choose from a variety of vegetables, such as cauliflower, sweet potato, rapini, kale, spinach, arugula, Swiss chard, bok choy, broccoli, Brussels sprouts, dandelion, beets and beet greens. Variety is key. The fiber will keep you fuller longer, and the balanced variety of vitamins and minerals will enhance your energy, improve your skin and hair health and aid in detoxification. Choose at least one meal each day to fill 50 percent of your plate with green vegetables.

4. Eat protein at every meal, and don't skip breakfast.

Protein is a macronutrient that has powerful effects. Protein stimulates the metabolic rate—hurray for fat-burning! It will balance your blood sugar and prevent cravings by keeping insulin hormone levels in check. Protein may take anywhere from three to five hours to digest. This means your stomach stays fuller longer. When you eat protein-rich meals, you naturally eat less overall.

Healthy protein options at each meal include eggs, chia, quinoa, fish, chicken, nuts and seeds, Greek yogurt (higher in protein than regular plain yogurt), plant-based protein powder, hemp seeds, lentils, beans and green superfoods (see page 114).

Studies show that people who skip breakfast are more prone to belly fat because of the resulting increase in insulin. High insulin levels also increase your cravings for refined sugars and carbohydrates. Having a breakfast such as a metabolism-boosting smoothie that contains a healthy dose of protein truly sets the stage for a joyful day (see recipe on page 17).

5. Snack, but eat the *right* snacks and eat only when you are actually hungry.

When most people want a quick snack, they tend to grab fast-acting refined carbohydrates like cookies, crackers or chips. The drive for these foods is even more intense when you go longer than three or four hours without eating anything or when you skip a meal. The body is a very smart machine! It knows that refined carbs quickly convert to glucose (a form of sugar) in the body, hence making them the obvious choice for a burst of energy when the glucose supply gets low. This is exactly why you may find that, on those days you were too busy to have lunch at work, when you get home all you want to eat is carbs.

This perpetual habit comes at a cost to the body. When you continually eat unhealthy snacks, their excess sugar will eventually be converted to fat. Additionally, eating high-sugar snacks will spike insulin levels, which can lead to an imbalance in blood sugar and put you at risk of developing type 2 diabetes.

Make a point of including protein in your snacks. It keeps blood sugar levels in check and it keeps you satiated for a longer time. The same goes for good fats. In other words, good fat and protein shut your belly up!

Now, I don't want you to go thinking that carbohydrates are bad. Carbs are not bad at all. In fact, they are essential for energy, fiber and nutrients. But not all carbs are created equally. Make sure you choose good carbs rather than bad carbs, as discussed in chapter 2.

Joyous Tip

Listen to your body, and snack only when you are actually hungry: If you eat a balanced meal for breakfast and find that you are not hungry two or three hours later, don't force yourself to eat a snack. Listen to your body. When you feel the warm sensation of hunger in your belly, then it's time to eat. Keep in mind that stress can alter your appetite hormones. Solution: Reduce stress, listen to your body's hunger cues and power-snack.

Here are some balanced snack suggestions:

- 5 to 10 small brown rice crackers with 2 tbsp (30 mL) nut butter and a sprinkle of cinnamon

- ¼ cup (60 mL) Superfood Trail Mix (page 215)

- 1 soft-boiled egg with cut-up veggies

- 1 cup (250 mL) cut-up veggies with 2 tbsp (30 mL) hummus

- 2 tbsp (30 mL) chocolate protein powder mixed with 1 cup (250 mL) almond milk

- 1 apple with 1 tbsp (15 mL) almond butter

- Half an avocado sprinkled with hemp seeds on some high-fiber crackers

- Chocolate Mint Pudding (page 270)

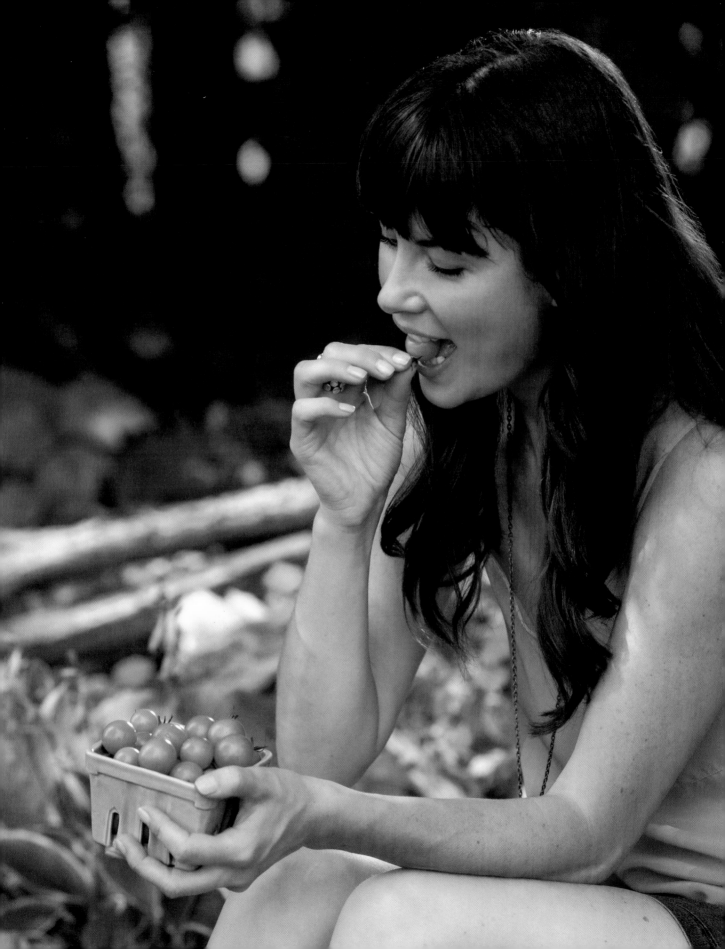

6. Keep a wellness journal.

For one week, write down everything you eat and drink. Studies show that keeping a food journal helps you reach your goals.

You'll find a food and wellness journal at the back of this book that you can photocopy. Record not only what you eat and drink but also how you feel. This will increase your awareness of your feelings toward food and yourself. Becoming aware helps you to break old habits that do not serve you well and create new ones that make you feel joyous inside and out.

My philosophy is that you do not need to count your calories or measure your food—let your inner wisdom be your guide. Free yourself from a need to put a number on everything food related! By keeping a food and wellness journal, you will become accustomed to listening to your body and giving it what it needs. The journal will also help you identify where your strengths and weaknesses are. Then you can take positive steps each week to improve in the areas that need a little more attention.

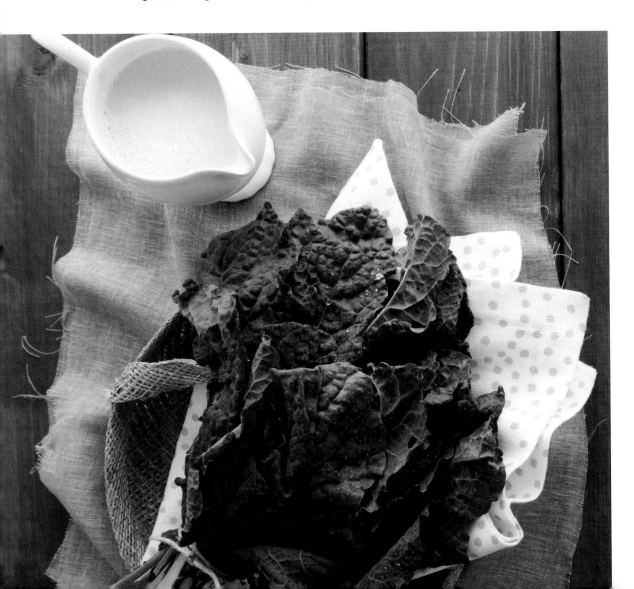

Metabolism-Booster Breakfast Smoothie

Rejuvenate and recharge your body and mind with an all-time favorite breakfast of mine. It's not only ideal as an energizing breakfast, but well balanced as a post-workout smoothie too. It combines a blend of complex carbs, lean protein and good fats to keep you satisfied, energized and balanced. Plus, it's darn tasty!

Makes 1 to 2 smoothies

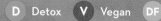 **D** Detox　**V** Vegan　**DF** Dairy-free　**GF** Gluten-free

1 banana, cut in chunks

1 cup (250 mL) fresh or
　frozen dark berries

1 cup (250 mL) spinach or kale leaves

1 cup (250 mL) unsweetened almond,
　brown rice, oat or hemp milk
　(rotate your nut milks each week)

2 tbsp (30 mL) whole chia seeds

1 tsp (5 mL) pure vanilla extract
　(or 2 or 3 drops of liquid stevia)

1 scoop plant-based protein powder

Filtered water and ice

Place all ingredients in your blender and purée for 30 to 60 seconds. Add filtered water to reach desired consistency.

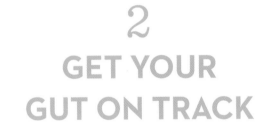

2

GET YOUR
GUT ON TRACK

On the Joyous Health wellness evaluation form that all my clients complete when they first come to me, there is a section that asks them to list three health goals or areas of concern. Nearly 80 percent of people give weight loss as the number-one reason they want assistance—even if they don't actually need to lose any. More often than not, the second goal is to deflate their belly bloat, and the third goal is often to have glowing, dewy skin.

But guess what? Weight loss, better digestion (bye-bye, bloated belly) and glowing skin are merely side effects of good health and a finely tuned digestive system—a joyous belly.

In this chapter, you'll learn all about your gut and become a certified joyous poo-ologist. I will share nutritionist-tested solutions to your most common (and perhaps most embarrassing) digestive problems. Most important, you will learn that it's not just what you eat but also what you assimilate, absorb and eliminate—or don't eliminate—that makes you *you*.

But first, let's take a tour through your digestive system so you get to know it a bit better.

. . .

A healthy gut equals a vibrant,
sexy, joyous body and mind.

. . .

Your Brain: The Control Center

The sound, sight, smell and texture of food send signals to the brain to prepare the gut to receive that food. Just chopping your veggies starts your digestive juices flowing. You start to salivate, and digestive enzymes and hormones begin to prepare your body to receive food. This is why, if you really want to improve your digestion, you should prepare your own meals instead of getting fast food. Another bonus is that when you make your own food, you tend to eat healthier because you have complete control of what you put on your plate. So be mindful when you are preparing food. Allow all your senses to be submerged in the wonderful art of food preparation and strengthen that digestive fire!

Your Mouth: The Chomper

Your stomach doesn't have teeth, so chew, chew, chew your food until it's a mushy paste. Can you hear your grandmother scolding you right now? "Chew your food, chew your food!" she would say. She had a point, and I'm on her side.

Most people chew a few times, swallow big chunks of food and chase them down with liquid. This is not a good way to eat! It's not a very kind thing to do to your digestive system and can lead to constipation, a slow-moving gut and poor absorption of nutrients. And if you don't properly absorb the nutrients from the food you eat, how can your body create cellular energy, or energy to play with your kids, or garden or walk the dog?

How do you know you've chewed enough? Think of an apple. You should chew it until you can no longer distinguish between the peel and the flesh.

Your saliva contains an enzyme called salivary amylase that starts to break down a small percentage of starches in the mouth as soon as you start chewing. Chewing your food to a mushy paste actually eases the burden on later stages of the digestive process. Digestive enzymes can work only on the surface of pieces of food. Because chewing increases the surface area of the food you eat, those digestive enzymes can get right into every nook and cranny in that piece of apple, and your body will better absorb the nutrients from it.

Isn't it just incredible how something as simple as properly chewing your food can improve your energy and enable you to do more of the things you love to do?

Remember the mindful-eating exercise in chapter 1? Chewing is a wonderful opportunity to indulge in some mindful eating.

SPIT OUT THE GUM!

I'm against gum chewing, and for a good reason. If you're a gum chewer, do you ever wonder why you're gassy and bloated and you perhaps even fart a lot? When you chew gum, your brain signals to your gut to prepare for food to come down the pipe. You start producing digestive juices, including stomach acids and enzymes. But of course nothing comes into your stomach because you are only chewing gum—you are tricking your body!

The result? You can deplete your digestive enzymes and lower your stomach acid, so that when you actually do eat food, your digestive fire is low, and as a result, you may have digestive problems such as gas and bloating. Besides that, the artificial sweeteners used in most gum are a whole other evil story and should be avoided at all costs (see page 74).

One of my first clients, "Sarah," was, at twenty-eight years old, a perfect example of the negative effects of gum chewing. Even though she was eating a good diet with lots of variety, she was constantly bloated. After reviewing her food journal and discussing her lifestyle (she had very little stress), I was baffled why she was always bloated. Then I uncovered something. Sarah was a real estate agent, and she worried about having bad breath, so she was constantly chewing gum. I advised her to stop immediately, and I gave her other advice for preventing bad breath (including taking probiotics, using a tongue brush and getting her gut health on track). As soon as she ditched the gum-chewing habit, she was bloat-free. Sarah was over the moon with joy because she was soon able to fit into her skinny jeans once again.

Your Stomach: The High-Powered Blender

So you've chewed, chewed and chewed some more. Now you swallow the food, and muscle contractions called peristalsis move it down your esophagus until it ends up in the digestive system's very own blender, your stomach. There, it is further sliced and diced (pulverized by peristalsis), then liquefied into a soupy substance called chyme.

Protein digestion occurs in the stomach when chemicals found in gastric juices, primarily hydrochloric acid, or HCl, and the enzyme pepsin, break apart protein chains made up of amino acids. These amino acids are the building blocks of life because they make up every single cell in your body. What happens in the stomach is therefore a crucial stage of digestion.

HCl is a strong acid—if dropped on your kitchen table, it would burn a hole in it. This extreme acidity explains why it does a great job killing microbes that are in the food you eat. But don't worry, your stomach is protected from acid damage by a thick lining of mucus.

The stomach usually takes between three and five hours to complete its job (three if you ate a light meal and five if your meal was heavy in the protein and fat department). After this, the stomach passes the soupy chyme along to the small intestine, where most of the digestion and absorption of nutrients occurs.

Your Liver: The Chemical Factory

As a nutritionist, I talk about this organ extensively in my seminars because our liver has 561 known functions, making it one of the hardest-working organs in the body.

I call it the chemical factory because toxic substances and waste products that are either taken in and absorbed by the intestines or produced by your body as a byproduct of metabolism are all detoxified in the liver. From alcohol to cigarette smoke, from foods with chemical additives to lotions you slather on your skin, all must be detoxified so they do not harm your body. Your liver takes these potentially harmful substances and neutralizes them, preparing them for elimination.

When your body is overburdened with chemicals and the liver cannot fully perform its job, you may suffer from allergies, low immune system function, skin disorders, hormonal imbalance and weight gain. That is why it's critical that you ease the chemical burden on your liver by drinking plenty of water to assist in the removal of these toxins and by eating detoxifying foods that contain liver-supporting nutrients.

The liver is also a major storage site for many of the nutrients absorbed through the wall of the small intestine. These nutrients include vitamins A, C, D, E, K and B_{12}, the minerals copper and iron, and glycogen, a form of energy. The liver also regulates glucose metabolism, releasing glucose as it is needed for energy.

From a Chinese medicine perspective, the liver holds a lot of emotional garbage, too. Practitioners of traditional Chinese medicine say that the liver stores anger and sadness and cannot function joyfully if you've not dealt with your emotions. Emotional wellness is a key factor in achieving your most joyous health.

Clearly, your liver works very hard and needs a lot of love. Enjoying the recipes provided in this book will give your liver the support it needs to help it carry out one of its most important functions, detoxification. Try the Detox Juice on page 174.

Your Small Intestine: Where the Magic Happens

The intestinal wall has two extremely important functions: (1) it allows nutrients such as vitamins and minerals to be absorbed into the bloodstream, and (2) it blocks foreign substances from entering your bloodstream. These foreign substances include chemicals, bacteria and other large molecules found in food. (Remember: chew, chew, chew! It makes this stage of digestion easier.) However, some medications or a poor diet can thin the lining of this wall, causing your gut to absorb substances that may be harmful. This is known as leaky gut syndrome, and it can lead to skin problems such as acne and eczema, as well as to food sensitivities and other health issues that can have a whole host of unpleasant effects.

Your small intestine is made up of three parts: the duodenum, jejunum and ileum. Each part absorbs different nutrients that help keep your cells joyous. Minerals are absorbed in the duodenum; protein, water-soluble vitamins and carbohydrates predominantly in the jejunum; and fat-soluble vitamins, cholesterol, fat and bile salts in the ileum. It is important that all three parts of the small intestine function efficiently for good digestion.

Your Large Intestine (Colon): The Grand Finale

It may be last, but it is certainly not least. After your small intestine has absorbed all the nutrients it can, your large intestine is the last stop in the digestive process before waste leaves your body. The average person can have anywhere from 7 to 25 pounds (3 to 11 kg) of impacted fecal matter in their gut. That's a lot of poop, but to put it in perspective, the digestive tract, from mouth to anus, is 25 to 35 feet (7.5 to 10.5 m) long, and if you were to stretch and flatten out just your small intestine, it would cover the entire surface of a tennis court!

The contents of your fecal matter are mainly fiber (the undigested material from plant foods), indigestible waste material, water and billions of naturally occurring bacteria. Each of these plays a key role in efficient digestion.

Fiber is absolutely essential because it helps to fill out the colon, absorbs toxins and waste, softens your poop and eases waste excretion. Bacteria—known as our gut flora—do wonderful things in your colon. Not only do they break down some previously undigested materials, but they also act on food residues to make vitamin K and biotin. Water mixes with the fecal mass to help it pass more easily from the body. Excess water is then reabsorbed into the body to prevent dehydration.

There's a lot going on, from the mouth onward! And when the pipes are working effectively, you detoxify and eliminate toxins regularly. If you don't have good digestion, though, these toxins try to escape in other ways. The leaky gut syndrome mentioned earlier, which can cause blemishes on your beautiful face or eczema on your hands, is an example of those toxins trying to escape out the wrong exits.

DANA'S STORY

One of my first clients, "Dana," had slim arms and legs, yet she had a very distended belly. She was exercising regularly, but she told me she was chronically constipated and became progressively bloated throughout the day. By the end of the day she always had to undo the top button of her pants. Bloating isn't much fun, especially when you wear suits to work every day and they are tight and uncomfortable by five o'clock.

After reviewing Dana's food journal and assessing her current state of health and her health history, I put her on a detox plan. I removed from her diet all common foods that cause sensitivity symptoms, increased her intake of fiber-rich foods, started her on a supplementation plan that involved digestive enzymes specific to her needs and had her take a high-dose probiotic.

We also focused on strategies to lower her stress levels. To replace her intensive bootcamp sessions three or four times a week, Dana committed herself to one or two classes a week at a local yoga studio. I also taught her alternate nostril breathing (see page 59) to help her relax whenever she felt stressed at work. Dana was extremely determined to change, and in four weeks, she lost a whopping 10 pounds.

Dana told me the biggest change was that she was now having regular, well-formed, detoxifying bowel movements once or twice a day—in her words, the kind of bowel movements that make you feel like you've lost five pounds and that flatten your belly. Not only did her tummy look flat, she had so much more energy.

When your gut is full of impacted fecal matter like Dana's was, toxins can be reabsorbed into the body, which may weaken your immune system, give you a foggy brain, lower your energy, make you feel puffy and affect the health of your skin.

After Dana and I had worked together for nearly three months, her friends were telling her how much younger she looked because the puffiness was gone from her face and she was simply glowing. She felt like a brand-new person.

Solutions to Common Digestive Problems: The Suffering Can End!

North America and many countries around the world are facing an epidemic of digestive illnesses directly related to the foods we eat (and don't eat) and the way we live our lives.

TV commercials commonly show a stressed-out person eating a burger and fries, then suffering from indigestion, which is temporarily relieved by an antacid or other heartburn drug. More than 80 or 90 million people suffer from digestive problems in North America every year, according to the Canadian Digestive Health Foundation and the US National Institute of Diabetes and Digestive and Kidney Diseases. Some of the most successful pharmaceutical drugs are the ever-popular antacids and over-the-counter laxatives. These drugs are making pharmaceutical manufacturers some of the wealthiest companies in the world.

Antacids work by weakening the hydrochloric acid in your stomach. Other heartburn drugs, such as H_2-receptor antagonists and proton-pump inhibitors, suppress the production of stomach acid. But do they really help? Are people getting better by popping a pill to prevent acid production? Is acid production even the problem in the first place? Perhaps not.

Every morsel you eat has the power to move you closer to health and further away from disease, or the opposite—closer and closer to illness. Unfortunately, too many people have simply accepted digestive illness as a fact of life and choose to suffer while popping pill after pill rather than dealing with the root cause of their symptoms. Instead of subscribing to the notion that a pill will fix you, acknowledge that your digestive problems offer an incredible opportunity for change. This is a blessing in disguise.

You have the power to heal your body with the way you live your life, the thoughts that you think, how often you move your body and the food you consume.

Based on what I hear from my clients and the types of over-the-counter digestive aids that have the strongest sales, these are the most common digestive complaints:

- constipation
- heartburn
- gas, flatulence and bloating
- irritable bowel syndrome

I will share solutions to get your gut back on track. Fortunately, there are simple and inexpensive solutions for any digestive concern. However, it is important that you seek the advice of your natural healthcare practitioner if your symptoms persist, since there are many natural solutions beyond this book that may benefit you and help bring your body back into balance.

Constipation

Straining to have a bowel movement, hard stools, rabbit-like pellets, infrequent or incomplete bowel movements, the feeling that your gut just is not emptied, having a bowel movement less than once a day—these are all hallmarks of constipation.

Constipation can lead to more issues than just a bloated belly. Constipation can cause

- allergies and skin problems, including eczema and acne
- fatigue
- headaches
- low energy
- mental fogginess
- moodiness
- pain and inflammation in the joints
- PMS

Constipation is a big problem. More than 27 percent of North Americans report feeling constipated, while in the United States alone, more than $875 million was spent on over-the-counter laxatives in 2011. That's a lot of people full of poop!

Many underlying factors may lead to constipation, including thyroid dysfunction, hormonal problems and certain medications. As well, some diseases can affect the body's ability to have a bowel movement, including Parkinson's disease, lupus, type 2 diabetes, kidney disease and colon cancer. It's best to rule out these possible causes by talking to your medical doctor. However, healthy digestion and good dietary habits may prevent all these chronic diseases from occurring in the first place.

Your bowel movements should be painless and effortless. The ideal stool should be chestnut brown, S-shaped and well formed. In a perfect world, you would be just like an infant and have a BM after every meal. However, with our busy lives, and the fact that we don't always have access to a washroom, having a BM after every meal may prove challenging. I recommend you aim to have one or two bowel movements each day. This means, of course, that you actually need to make time for this.

Even if you have one or two bowel movements each day, you may still be constipated or have a large amount of backed-up fecal matter, so it is important to check what's known as your bowel transit time.

Do the Beet Test

Buy some raw beets, wash them and peel off the skin if they are not organic. Using a cheese grater or mandoline, grate the beets. Mix them into a salad or roast them and enjoy with some extra-virgin olive oil and pepper. Better yet, make my Beet Goat Cheese Dip (page 222). Don't use jarred pickled beets from the grocery store. They won't have the same effect because the red pigment, called betalaine, has likely been destroyed during processing.

After you've eaten the beets, look in the toilet after each bowel movement and take note when you see a red color in your stools. Do not be alarmed! This can be quite shocking the first time you see it. You may also notice your urine turns pinkish or red, a phenomenon called beeturia.

The optimal bowel transit time is twelve to twenty-four hours. However, some of my clients have reported not seeing red stools until four or five days later. This means the same food has been sitting in their gut for up to 120 hours!

If that doesn't seem like a big deal to you, imagine a glass of full-fat cream sitting on a picnic table in the summer for four or five days. What will happen to it? It starts to rot—it grows bacteria and mold. That's not something you would want to drink, is it? Your gut is like that glass of cream. It's a warm environment full of yeast and bacteria (both good and bad). When food sits in your gut for a long time, it does the same thing as that glass of cream. It begins to rot, and the bacteria and yeast feed off it, potentially producing toxic byproducts and causing gas and bloating, which make constipation worse and can create other problems down the line.

When fecal matter sits too long in the gut, reabsorption of cholesterol, hormones and waste products can occur. This is why constipation can lead to high cholesterol and hormonal imbalances like PMS. Constipation means more than just having a bloated belly!

So, how are you going to get your gut moving to ensure you are not full of twenty-five pounds of poop? The top natural solutions for reducing constipation are:

- drinking more water
- eating more fiber-rich and water-dense foods
- reducing stress
- increasing or reducing consumption of certain foods
- taking a probiotic supplement

Drink More Water

Our bodies are made up of more than 70 percent water. Every cell is dependent on water to help push nutrients in and pull waste products out for elimination. Water is vital for our survival; we cannot live without it. Even mild dehydration that hasn't even reached the point of triggering thirst can result in headaches and low energy. The simple habit of drinking more water is absolutely essential for a healthy digestive system and the elimination of toxins.

Your gut is a water-rich environment. In fact, when you are dehydrated, the first place your kidneys will signal the body to take up water from is the large intestine, so that vital functions such as the ability of your heart to pump blood can be maintained. This means that your large intestine can easily become dehydrated, making your stools dry and difficult to pass.

HOW MUCH WATER SHOULD YOU BE DRINKING?

There is a no one-size-fits-all answer. For example, for each cup of coffee or other caffeinated beverage you drink, you need to drink one glass (approximately 2 cups/500 mL) of water just to break even, because caffeine is a diuretic. If you exercise often and sweat a lot, you will need to increase your water consumption as well. On the other hand, if you don't drink coffee and you eat a lot of hydrating foods such as raw fruits and vegetables, then you don't need to be chugging back twelve glasses of water every day.

Aim for at least six to eight glasses of water or herbal tea per day (assuming a glass to be 1 to 2 cups/250 to 500 mL). Beyond this, a good way to gauge your hydration needs is to look at the color of your urine. Assuming you are not on any supplements or medications that change the color of your urine, it should be pale yellow. Bright yellow indicates urine that is too concentrated, and therefore you are likely dehydrated. Completely clear urine means that you may be drinking too much water, which can actually be hard on your kidneys.

The best way to start your day, as mentioned in chapter 1, is with a large glass of filtered water (1⅔ to 2 cups/400 to 500 mL) with a squeeze of lemon or a splash of apple cider vinegar. Lemon or cider vinegar with water helps to stimulate a bowel movement because it strengthens the liver and improves your digestive fire, which helps to move waste products through more efficiently.

Eat More Fiber-Rich and Water-Dense Foods

This is likely something you've heard before. The good news is that the majority of recipes in this book provide more than enough daily fiber. Fiber, or roughage, adds bulk to the stool and helps the body eliminate toxins.

Fiber helps to strengthen the gut muscles, which improves peristalsis, the action that moves food through your digestive system. When you eat "lazy," low-fiber foods such as white pasta, white rice and white bread, your gut becomes lazy too, and constipation is often a result. Fiber also acts as a scrub, brushing away wastes from the colon wall, and as a sponge, absorbing potentially harmful toxins and chemicals.

Increase your consumption of fiber slowly, as a sudden increase in the amount of roughage can irritate the gut, causing gas and bloating. It's just as important to cut back on foods that are low in fiber and water, including meat, cheese, white bread and sugary pastries, cookies, candies and cakes.

Aim to eat five to ten servings of fruits and vegetables every day, but do not feel limited to the foods listed above. The sky is the limit! For a more detailed list of fiber-rich foods, see page 42.

Most cases of constipation can be resolved naturally. Eating more fiber and drinking more water usually solve the problem fairly quickly.

MY FAVORITE FIBER-RICH, NUTRIENT-DENSE AND HYDRATING FOODS

- apples
- asparagus
- avocados
- broccoli
- Brussels sprouts
- cabbage
- cauliflower
- celery
- chia seeds
- kale
- pears
- sweet potatoes
- watermelon

Reduce Stress

Different kinds of stress have different effects on digestion. *Chronic* stress slows down digestion by impeding the stomach's performance. When you eat when you're under stress, do you ever feel like you have a brick in your gut? That's stress in action. *Acute* stress, on the other hand, can actually speed things up by prompting the gut to push waste products through too quickly, preventing adequate digestion and absorption of nutrients.

Remember, it's not only what you eat, it's also how you live your life that affects digestion. Reducing stress is absolutely essential for effective digestion.

When you are stressed, your nervous system is in "fight or flight" mode. The last thing your body wants to do right then is digest food. Your gut will either shut down digestion by inhibiting the secretion of stomach acid and digestive enzymes, leading to a very slow-moving gut, or do everything in its power to eliminate all the gut's contents, resulting in diarrhea.

Increase or Reduce Consumption of Certain Foods

EAT MORE OF THESE FOODS

- chia seeds and flaxseeds (sprouted are best)
- fermented foods such as raw sauerkraut, kefir, kombucha, organic tempeh (fermented soy)
- fiber-rich foods (see page 42)
- fresh fruit, especially pears, apples, peaches and dark berries
- good fats, including avocados, extra-virgin olive oil and flaxseed or hemp oil
- green superfoods such as spirulina (see chapter 5)
- herbal teas, especially dandelion licorice tea and nettle leaf tea
- leafy green vegetables such as kale, arugula, spinach and bok choy
- lemon and water (see page 12)
- sea vegetables, including arame, dulse, kombu and nori
- sprouted foods such as sunflower sprouts, pea sprouts, sprouted lentils and bean sprouts
- raw fruits and vegetables (introduce them slowly if you are not currently eating many raw foods)
- real "whole" grains such as quinoa, brown rice, millet, amaranth, teff, buckwheat, kamut, oats and spelt

EAT LESS OF THESE FOODS

- red meat
- dairy products
- sugary treats and sweets
- white flour products and white rice
- genetically modified foods such as corn, soy and wheat
- dried fruits (or rehydrate them in filtered water before consuming)
- commercial cereals and protein bars (they can be full of additives and preservatives that slow your gut down—I like to call them "cement" in your colon)

Finally, if there is any food that you have been eating every day for longer than four to six weeks, cut it out of your diet for two weeks. You can become sensitive to the foods you eat most often, so eliminating them for a short while will help you rule out food sensitivities.

Take a Probiotic Supplement

Probiotics can be your best friend. *Pro* means "for" and *biotics* means "life," so probiotics are the good bacteria (the bugs) in your body. I'm not saying that taking a pill is a cure-all, but probiotics are one of the most well-researched supplements for digestive health and they are particularly helpful for constipation.

Did you know that your digestive system is home to more than 100 trillion bacteria—a billion of those in your mouth, and most of the rest in your small intestine and colon? In fact, you have more bacteria in your gut than cells in your entire body. According to Elizabeth Lipski, author of *Digestive Wellness*, the dry weight of your stool consists of 80 percent bacteria, and half of that is still alive. The balance of good versus bad bacteria is absolutely critical for healthy digestion, your immune system, vitamin and mineral absorption and much more.

From person to person, the type of digestive bacteria, or gut flora, can differ drastically based on diet. In general, those who eat high-fiber foods, including lots of fruits and vegetables, and less meat have a better ratio of good to bad bacteria than people who eat the typical Western diet full of refined carbohydrates, sugar and food additives.

Antibiotics, birth control pills and corticosteroid drugs can further alter the delicate balance of good bacteria to bad bacteria. When bad bacteria get out of hand, the most common result is an overgrowth of a yeast called *Candida*. *Candida* can cause a whole host of problems, from acne and itchy skin to yeast infections in the mouth and vagina. It may even enter the bloodstream, causing systemic candidiasis.

Digestive bacteria are a hot topic in the news, and there's no shortage of probiotic products, from yogurts to ice creams, popping up on grocery store shelves everywhere. So what's all the fuss about? Well, the good bacteria do an absolutely incredible job of keeping us healthy and keeping the bad bacteria in check.

- They keep our immune system strong and play an important role in our ability to fight infectious disease. For example, *Lactobacillus acidophilus*, found in fermented dairy products such as yogurt, increases the activity of immune system fighters, including macrophages and lymphocytes.

- They prevent or increase resistance to food poisoning. *L. acidophilus* inhibits up to twenty-six different bacteria that make us sick, from *E. coli* to *Salmonella*.

- They make biotin, folic acid and vitamins B_1, B_2, B_3, B_5, B_6, B_{12} and K.

- They increase absorption of calcium, copper, iron, magnesium and manganese.

- They manufacture substances that can assist in lowering our risk of disease and cancer.

- They help relieve inflammatory bowel diseases, constipation, diarrhea, etc.

- They help us digest lactose. Some people can tolerate yogurt but not milk for the simple reason that there is more good bacteria in yogurt.

- They aid in treating vaginal yeast infections, thrush, urinary tract infections and arthritis and may positively affect cholesterol levels.

- Recent research shows they even impact your brain function, including preventing anxiety and depression.

The two most abundant groups of flora are lactobacilli, found in the small intestine, and bifidobacteria, found primarily in the colon. Here's the deal: we are born with a sterile digestive tract. We are then exposed to good bacteria in breast milk, and with every breath and touch, bacteria enter the body to colonize and make a cozy home. (Breast-fed babies have increased numbers of *Lactobacillus* and *Bifidobacterium* species from mama—yet another reason to breast-feed your baby.) Within the first few days of life, we become home to hundreds of bacteria. Often, when babies are unable to properly colonize the friendly bacteria, they become irritable and colicky, they have gas and they may even have eczema on their bottom. They are also more susceptible to allergies and asthma, according to Elizabeth Lipski.

Unfortunately, the friendly bacteria are only a small percentage of our total bacteria. Most disease-causing bacteria thrive at human body temperature, and a fever kills them by overheating your body. (Don't you just love how smart your body is?) If you have a sudden invasion of *Salmonella* bacteria, your body reacts quickly, trying to eliminate them via a sudden bout of diarrhea, vomiting and possibly even a fever. Be thankful for this response! I cringe at the thought of people taking diarrhea-suppressing drugs when they have food poisoning, as this could lead to more health complications down the road. The last thing you want to do is plug yourself up and keep those bad bacteria inside you.

You can boost the number of good flora by eating them: kefir, yogurt (if you don't have a dairy sensitivity), sauerkraut, tempeh, miso, kimchi and kombucha are excellent sources. As well, avoid processed foods and chlorinated water, reduce stress and take a good-quality probiotic supplement. There is an array of probiotic supplements on the market. Every one of us has slightly different needs, so it is important that you first speak with a practitioner to find out what is best for you.

As Dr. Bernard Jensen has stated many times in his books, your gut health determines the health of your entire body. Keeping your gut healthy with good bacteria is absolutely critical to the health of your whole body. I'm not saying that probiotics solve every problem, but they are certainly one of the most basic supplements that most people would benefit from taking.

Heartburn

I am very familiar with heartburn, which has been persistent in my family for years. Acid reflux, gastroesophageal reflux disease (GERD), over-production of acid—whatever you call it, it's not fun, and it's a complaint I commonly hear in the initial session with my clients.

Ironically, the majority of people who complain of heartburn actually don't produce *enough* stomach acid. Heartburn is more often than not a result of improper food combining (for example, eating a steak and mashed potatoes together may be a recipe for poor digestion), drinking too many liquids with meals, a poor ratio of good to bad bacteria, overeating, eating too late in the evening, a poor diet or stress.

Before you go taking any pills to suppress acid production, consider these points.

- Acid-suppressing medications can create an overly alkaline stomach environment. But minerals require an acidic digestive environment to be properly digested and absorbed. This is when that glass of lemon and water comes in handy! Even though lemon juice promotes an alkaline body, it strengthens the digestive fire, which means food will be more effectively moved through the body. If you lack proper stomach acid, you don't absorb your minerals, and this can contribute to type 2 diabetes, some cancers, chronic pain, arthritis and even heart problems.

- Stomach acid is needed for the proper breakdown of proteins into amino acids. Amino acids are the building blocks of life. Every cell in your entire body depends on amino acids, from your skin cells to your brain cells. For example, without the proper breakdown and absorption of amino acids, your neurotransmitters—brain chemicals—do not have the raw materials to function.

- Stomach acid is one of the first lines of defense against pathogenic, or disease-causing, bacteria. A lack of stomach acid can mean more bad bacteria getting in through the digestive tract, leading to food poisoning, other illnesses and disease.

TWO SIMPLE STOMACH ACID TESTS

1. BAKING SODA TEST

This test will help give you a sense of whether you have too much or too little stomach acid. First thing in the morning, on an empty stomach, drink ¼ tsp (1 mL) of baking soda stirred into 1 cup (250 mL) of water. Time how long it takes to burp. If you haven't burped within five minutes, stop timing. Do the test four days in a row and record your results. When you drink baking soda, you create a chemical reaction in your stomach between the baking soda and the hydrochloric acid. The result is carbon dioxide gas, which makes you burp. If you have low stomach acid, it will take you longer than three minutes to burp. If you have adequate stomach acid, you will burp within the first two or three minutes.

2. BETAINE HCL CHALLENGE TEST

To complete this test, you will need to purchase a bottle of 650 mg Betaine HCl containing pepsin at a health food store. Note: Anti-inflammatory medications such as NSAIDs, corticosteroids and aspirin increase the chances of ulcers in the stomach, and Betaine HCl can further increase the risk of gastritis. Consult a natural healthcare practitioner before trying this test or supplementing.

1. Prepare a high-protein meal with at least 6 ounces (170 g) of meat, chicken or fish.

2. In the middle of the meal, take one capsule of Betaine HCl.

3. Finish your meal, and pay attention to your digestion.

If you don't notice any discomfort after your meal or any improvement in your digestion, it is very likely that your stomach acid is too low. If you start to feel a heaviness, burning or warmth, these are signs that you likely have adequate stomach acid. You can drink a mixture of ½ tsp (2 mL) of baking soda and 1 cup (250 mL) of water to stop any discomfort.

If two subsequent stomach acid tests indicate you have low acid, then you know your heartburn is not the result of too much acid. I have found this to be the case with the majority of people! Which of course raises the question, Why are so many people taking antacids and acid-suppressing medications they don't need?

Joyous Solutions to Heartburn

These suggestions not only help with heartburn but can be extremely beneficial for a variety of digestive problems.

Practice basic food combining. Food combining is a set of guidelines to follow when you are eating that reduce heartburn, increase bowel transit time and can be an effective weight loss tool—when you eliminate more effectively, you are less bloated and not full of pounds of poop.

Do not drink fluids while eating solids. Drinking while you eat dilutes your digestive fire and can also lead to bloating and gas. Drink liquids 20 to 30 minutes before a meal or 45 minutes after a meal. Puréed soups are the exception.

Eat fruit alone or first thing in the morning. Fruit tends to ferment easily after it's eaten, especially when it's eaten with protein and fat and when your digestion is weak. The gaseous byproducts of this fermentation get pushed up through the esophagus, promoting heartburn. You will notice that some recipes in this book include fruit with other foods. You may combine fruit with other foods if you do not suffer from heartburn or other digestive issues.

Eat from lightest to heaviest. This eases the burden of digestion. Protein digests mainly in the stomach, whereas carbohydrates digest mainly in the small intestine. Eat the lightest foods on your plate first—often the carbohydrates—and finish your meal with the heaviest foods, usually the proteins and fats.

Do not combine a high-starch food with a protein in the same meal. High-starch foods ferment easily and are mostly digested in the small intestine. For example, eating white potatoes with a steak is a recipe for digestive problems because the steak may take a few hours to leave the stomach while the potatoes digest quickly and may ferment.

Avoid eating dessert on a full stomach. Eat it on a near-empty stomach, not immediately after a meal, to prevent any fermentation.

Do not eat after 8 P.M. Your digestive fire slowly becomes weaker as the day progresses. If you must eat later, make sure you eat something that's easier to digest, such as a smoothie (page 164) as a meal replacement or Overnight Strawberry Chia Pudding (page 157), provided you've had an earlier snack, as the pudding may not be filling enough.

Drink lemon and water (page 12) every morning on an empty stomach.

Eliminate dairy and gluten for two weeks. Then reintroduce them one at a time and record any reaction in a food journal. Permanently eliminate the foods that cause heartburn.

Avoid overly spicy foods and overeating in general. Spicy foods can aggravate your gut, and when you overeat, gas pushes up through the esophagus because your stomach is overstuffed, causing pain.

Limit coffee, caffeine-containing beverages and fizzy drinks.

Drink helpful teas. These include peppermint, chamomile, slippery elm and ginger.

Try bitters. Consider using a bitter to stimulate good digestion before you eat. Some bitters worth trying are peppermint, calendula, dandelion, artichoke leaf, blessed thistle, angelica, motherwort, wormwood and bitter orange peel. These can be taken as a tea, tincture or capsule. You can also look for a "digestive bitter" at the health food store that has a combination of bitter ingredients in one formula.

Take digestion-supporting supplements.

- Betaine HCl (derived from beets). Take two 500-mg capsules with meals three times a day or as advised by your natural healthcare practitioner.

- probiotics (see page 31)

- digestive enzymes

- L-glutamine. If you've been suffering from heartburn for a few months or longer, you may find this amino acid helpful. It protectively coats your digestive tract, including your esophagus, and actually repairs damage to the lining of both the esophagus and the stomach. Take 5 g (about 2 tsp/10 mL) a day. It can also reduce sugar cravings, help with alcohol addiction and enhance the immune system.

Reduce stress. Do yoga, meditate, listen to relaxing music, take a bath. Reducing stress improves digestion.

Get enough sleep. Ensure you get at least eight hours of sleep in complete darkness.

Exercise. Move your beautiful booty every single day! Get your heart rate up for at least 15 to 20 minutes each day and increase to 45 minutes a day once you've adapted.

Gas, Flatulence and Bloating

Now and again, it's totally normal to pass gas or burp. But if this is a regular occurrence, then it's time to pay attention to what your body is telling you, as these are signs that something you're eating is not agreeing with you. Additionally, bad-smelling flatulence is a common sign that you may not be properly digesting gluten—a protein in wheat, rye and barley. It can even be a symptom of an autoimmune disease such as celiac disease.

Joyous Solutions to Gas, Flatulence and Bloating

- Eat mindfully. Take time to enjoy your meal to prevent overeating. (See page 6.)
- Eat slowly and chew, chew, chew your food until it is a paste. (See page 20.)
- Eat smaller meals, and eat only when you are actually hungry— when you feel that warm feeling in your stomach.
- Do not eat when you are stressed out.
- Follow the food combining suggestions on page 36.
- Drink lemon and water before a meal. (See page 12.)
- Include herbs such as ginger, peppermint, dill and fennel in your meals.
- Avoid chewing gum.

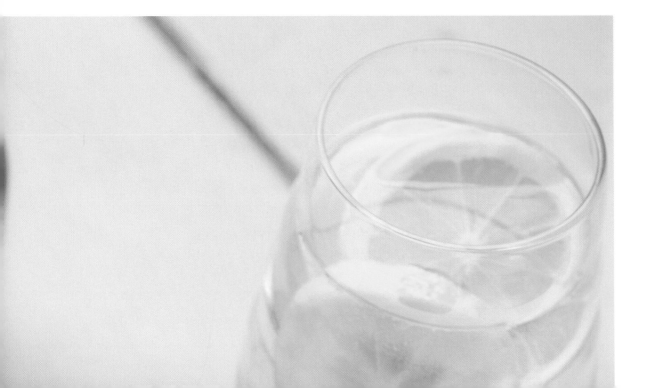

Irritable Bowel Syndrome

Irritable bowel syndrome, or IBS, is the medical name for a group of varied symptoms that occur together and affect the large intestine, including cramping, pain, constipation and diarrhea. IBS, though, tells us nothing about the root cause of these symptoms. It's important that you seek medical attention if you experience these symptoms because they could indicate a more serious problem, such as ulcerative colitis or Crohn's disease.

Two of the most common causes of IBS are stress and too much sugar. According to naturopath and author Dr. Michael Murray, "Stress increases the motility (the rhythmic contractions of the intestine that propel food through the digestive tract) of the colon and leads to abdominal pain and irregular bowel functions." On the other hand, refined sugar decreases intestinal motility and leads to constipation. Reducing both stress and sugar is absolutely essential when dealing with IBS!

Joyous Solutions to Irritable Bowel Syndrome

Reduce stress. Do yoga, meditate, listen to relaxing music or take a bath. Reducing stress lowers cortisol and adrenaline levels, stress hormones that both slow down the digestive system and exacerbate inflammation.

Ensure you get at least eight hours of sleep in complete darkness.

Eliminate the most common food allergens for two weeks, including dairy (especially cheese), gluten, corn, soy, peanuts and shellfish. Then reintroduce them one at a time and record any reaction in a food journal. Permanently eliminate the foods that cause a reaction.

Eliminate sugar and all foods containing refined sugars.

Eat fiber-rich foods to help with intestinal motility (see page 29). Fiber is especially helpful for those with constipation, but be sure to introduce it slowly and take note of how your body reacts.

Consider taking one of the following supplements:

- peppermint oil, in 100 mg capsule or liquid form, before meals to soothe the intestinal lining
- aloe vera juice, 1 tbsp (15 mL) before meals on an empty stomach
- a high-potency greens supplement that contains more than 1000 mg of spirulina (one scoop of Greens+ O in 2 cups/500 mL of water would be a great choice)

Eat Fiber

It is important to eat fiber-rich foods every day. Fiber provides the following health benefits:

- promotes regular bowel movements and prevents constipation
- supports healthy elimination and detoxification
- decreases hemorrhoids
- decreases the risk of colon and breast cancer
- lowers cholesterol and the risk of heart disease
- aids in weight loss and helps maintain healthy body weight
- normalizes blood sugar and reduces the risk of type 2 diabetes
- eliminates the need for laxatives, which may deplete minerals and dehydrate your body
- balances hormones by promoting the elimination of waste, including excess hormones in your bowel movements

Dietary Fiber

Dietary fiber is the indigestible material from plant foods. There are two types:

Insoluble fiber doesn't dissolve in water. By increasing the bulk of the stool, it helps move waste material through the colon faster. This is important for people who suffer from constipation or irregularity. Insoluble fiber has also been shown to lower blood sugar and decrease the risk of type 2 diabetes. Insoluble fiber is found in whole grains, wheat bran, nuts and many vegetables.

Soluble fiber absorbs water. It therefore softens stools, making them easier to eliminate from the body. Some soluble fibers bind to bile acids containing cholesterol and carry them out of the body, reducing the risk of heart disease. Soluble fiber is found in fruits, vegetables and grains, including apples, citrus fruits, oats, barley, flaxseeds, psyllium and legumes.

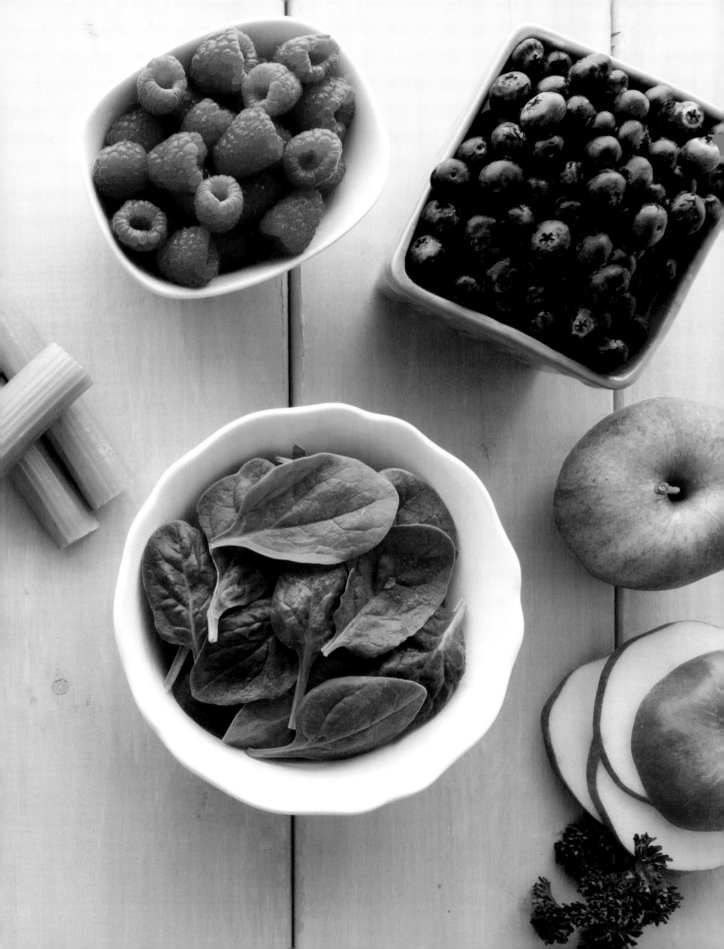

Top Fiber-Rich Foods

High-Fiber Vegetables

- broccoli
- Brussels sprouts
- cabbage
- carrots
- celery
- eggplant
- greens—spinach, collards, kale, turnip greens, beet greens
- mushrooms
- peas—black-eyed peas, green peas
- peppers
- potato with skin
- rhubarb
- squash
- sweet potato

High-Fiber Fruits

- apples
- avocado
- bananas
- berries—blueberries, blackberries, raspberries
- dried fruits—figs, raisins, apricots, dates, prunes
- grapefruit
- guava
- kiwi
- oranges
- pears

Other High-Fiber Foods

- beans and lentils
- chickpeas (garbanzo beans)
- nuts—almonds, brazil nuts, peanuts, walnuts, cashews
- seeds—chia, flax, pumpkin, sunflower

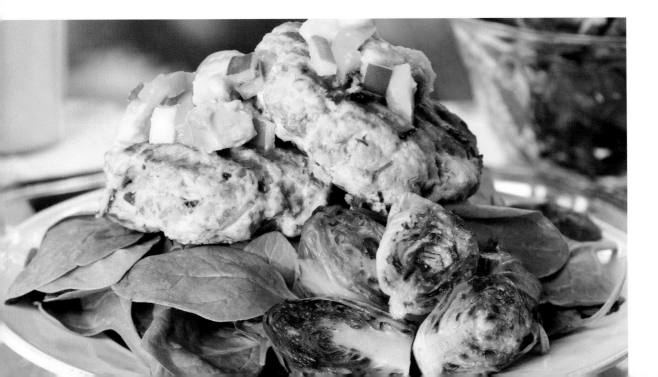

Anti-Bloat
Stomach-Calming Tea

We often get bloated because we improperly combine foods, which then end up putrefying in the gut and creating byproducts that make you bloated and can lead to heartburn. The lemon in this tea effectively strengthens the digestive fire by stimulating the production of bile and hydrochloric acid. In other words, it helps to strengthen the gut and deflate your belly bloat. Ginger is an excellent anti-inflammatory and can reduce any inflammation in the intestines. You can drink this tea before or after a meal or whenever you have a bellyache. Add some raw honey and you have a wonderful immune-boosting tea!

Makes 1 drink

D Detox **V** Vegan **DF** Dairy-free **GF** Gluten-free

Juice of ½ lemon
Chunk of peeled fresh ginger (about the size of your thumb)
1 cup (250 mL) filtered hot water

Place lemon juice and ginger in a mug. Pour hot water over lemon and ginger and let steep for a few minutes. Remove ginger and let tea cool slightly before drinking. Drinking the tea piping hot can damage the lining of your esophagus and the mucosal lining in your gut.

3
FOODS, SUPPLEMENTS AND HABITS FOR A JOYOUS MOOD

How you feed your body will affect your mood, and how you feel about your body will affect the foods you choose. You have choices!

The kind of day you have at work will influence your food choices, but you will have a better day at work if you choose good-mood foods rather than bad-mood foods that provide a temporary lift followed by a crash. Rather than getting caught up in a vicious cycle of eating bad-mood foods, feeling guilty about it and then depriving yourself, I want you to eat well, feel well and continue on a joyous path.

The knowledge that you gain in this chapter will provide you with a wonderful opportunity to harness the power you have within to choose joyous thoughts and good foods and keep you on the path to feeling your best!

. . .

When you take care of your body,
you will have a healthy and joyous
place to live for years to come.

. . .

Food and Your Mood

Have you ever noticed how a meal makes you feel ten minutes, thirty minutes, two hours or even half a day later? Do any of these scenarios sound familiar?

- You had a burger and fries and suddenly feel heavy and sluggish.

- You are flying high from that coffee or sugary snack, but three hours later, you are falling asleep at your desk from the blood sugar crash and ready for another hit.

- You had pizza and wings and now feel so gassy that you need to undo the top button of your jeans.

- You ate a bag of movie-theater popcorn, and the next day you feel sluggish and have a headache.

- You've been depriving yourself of food, and you feel moody and irritable and you have low energy.

These are examples of how food can change your mood. What if you could always eat foods that energize you and make you feel joyous? Well, you can! And it really is that easy to improve your mood! The key is to be aware of how particular foods make you feel.

The best way to track the food–mood connection is to keep a food and wellness journal, writing down what you are eating, how you feel at the time and any negative effects afterwards. (You'll find a journal on page 276.) The journal will help you become aware of how different foods make you feel. You will begin to notice the emotions surrounding what you eat, and begin to see why you eat these foods in the first place.

Many of us today are disconnected from what we eat. We eat more fast food and processed food, and so we have much less involvement in the creation of our food, and we even discount the food–mood connection. This is why food journaling, as described in chapter 1, can be an effective way to make us aware of how food affects us.

How Mood Affects Your Food Choices

Always remember that food is not going to solve your problems. Figure out what's eating you, rather than eating your feelings. Do any of these scenarios sound familiar?

- You've had a crappy day at work and you are ready for two heaping servings of your favorite macaroni and cheese.

- You had a fight with your significant other and you are ready to get snuggly with that pint of ice cream.

- You are flying high. You just got a big promotion at work and are ready for a night of indulgence and alcohol.

- You had a really stressful day and are ready to escape with a bottle of wine.

- You feel depressed, so you eat chocolate bars and candy to feel good.

What if there were ways to improve your mood that did not involve food? What if you dealt with the issues that made you stressed, got you down or upset you without using food? There *are* other solutions, and I'll share them with you in this chapter. But first, let's talk about how hormones can affect your mood.

Mood Hormones

The mood you experience at any given time is related to the events of your day, the health of your body and, in small part, your genetic makeup.

Both the events of your day and the health of your body are entirely under your control. True, the events of your day may have caused you to feel stressed, but stress is simply your reaction to a situation. You have the power to be entirely responsible for your reaction. That means you have the power to let a crappy day put you in a funk for the rest of the evening—or not. It is your choice. Isn't that amazing?

Neurotransmitters—which are hormones—are responsible for feelings of happiness, motivation, joy, anxiety, anger and sadness. The three main mood neurotransmitters are dopamine, norepinephrine and serotonin. And then there is the queen bee of neurotransmitters, nitric oxide (not to be confused with laughing gas). According to Dr. Christiane Northrup, author of *Women's Bodies, Women's Wisdom*, not only does nitric oxide increase the circulation of blood throughout the entire body, it also has the ability to balance out serotonin and dopamine. Nitric oxide is produced when you exercise, have sex, meditate or think joyful and loving thoughts—proof positive that creating joyful events during your day will improve your mood and well-being.

The health of your body and its neurotransmitters also depends upon the vitamins, minerals, proteins and essential fatty acids you eat daily. If you chronically eat a crappy diet, then you will be lacking in the nutrients essential for creating a happy mood in the first place. If you continue on this path, you may find yourself on an emotional rollercoaster day after day and wondering why your life is such a mess.

I'm not saying that food is the answer to everything, but food is a good place to start when you don't feel your most joyous self. It's something you do have power over.

Food Allergies and Sensitivities

As the old saying goes, One man's food is another man's poison. That simply means that different people can have very different reactions to exactly the same food.

Beyond hormones, food allergies are another reason food can put you in a bad mood. For example, if you have a sensitivity to gluten, as millions of North Americans do, it could be the cause of the headache and low energy that make you feel frustrated and unhappy—after eating pizza the night before. You don't have to be allergic to a food to be sensitive to it.

The top food allergens, according to Health Canada, are as follows:

- eggs
- milk
- mustard
- peanuts
- seafood (fish, crustaceans and shellfish)
- sesame
- soy
- sulfites (preservatives in dried fruit and naturally occurring in wine)
- tree nuts
- wheat

The majority of health problems associated with food sensitivities are described as "delayed onset." This means their symptoms do not manifest immediately. In fact, according to naturopath Dr. Michael Murray, up to 80 percent of food sensitivities produce symptoms that show up two hours to several days after you've eaten the food. That wheat cereal with skim milk you ate on Monday morning could be what's making you sluggish and moody on Tuesday.

If you suspect a bad-mood food after recording a food journal, remove the food for two weeks and re-evaluate how you feel.

Joyous Mood Foods and Nutrients

These are the top nutrients that can support a joyous mood.

Good Carbohydrates

Good carbohydrates are called complex carbohydrates, as opposed to refined carbohydrates. They're called "good" because they do all of the following (beyond just promoting a joyous mood):

- provide rich sources of nutrients, such as A, C, B-complex and E vitamins, and minerals such as selenium, iron, magnesium and potassium

- provide the body with long-lasting energy and replace glycogen stores in your muscles and liver

- keep your metabolism functioning efficiently

- keep cravings for sweets and salty snacks at bay and stabilize your mood by balancing your blood sugar

- lower cholesterol because they are a rich source of fiber

- help build lean muscle tissue by providing nutrients to aid in growth and development

- provide a slow release of glucose that gives the brain sustained energy and regulates mood

- are essential for the production of serotonin

SOURCES OF GOOD CARBS

Whole Grains

- amaranth
- barley
- brown rice
- bulgur
- kamut
- millet
- oats
- rye
- spelt
- wheat
- wild rice

Beans

- black
- garbanzo
- kidney
- navy
- pinto

Other Sources

- chia seeds
- flaxseeds
- psyllium
- fruits (all types, fresh or frozen)
- vegetables (all types, fresh or frozen)

Joyous Tip

Be cautious of "whole wheat" and "whole grain" breads. In Canada, food manufacturers are allowed to remove 5 percent of the wheat kernel—which translates to 70 percent of the germ, where most of the nutrients are found—and still call the product "whole wheat."

Even if a product is labeled "whole grain," you still need to be careful. In Canada, the term "whole grain" means that the product must contain 100% of the wheat kernel, unlike products labeled "whole wheat." But where it gets tricky is when a "whole grain" bread contains only small amounts of these whole grains and is otherwise full of refined flour products. Read the whole ingredients list carefully.

High-Quality Protein

Protein is not only a building block of neurotransmitters but it also helps keep your blood sugar balanced and your mood in check. When you eat some protein together with your carbs, it slows the release of glucose, a form of sugar, into the bloodstream. This provides your brain with a steady supply of glucose rather than the short burst followed by a crash that refined carbs and a meal lacking protein can cause.

As discussed in chapter 1, protein is essential not only at breakfast and for power snacks but also at lunch and dinner. Any meal you eat should include a high-quality protein if you want to receive the benefit of a joyous mood.

Joyous Tip

Include protein in your snack or meal. Protein promotes fat-burning! It also keeps insulin levels in check. High insulin = increased belly fat storage.

- beans and lentils (sprouted*)
- beef (lean and organic)
- chia seeds
- chicken (organic)
- eggs (whole)
- fish
- Greek yogurt (organic)
- hemp products
  (seeds and protein powders)
- nuts and nut butters
- plant-based protein powders
- seeds and seed butters
- spirulina

* Sprouted beans and lentils have higher levels of vitamins (especially the B-complex vitamins) and protein content, and they are more digestible than unsprouted legumes. If beans make you gassy, you are not digesting them properly. Be sure to follow the cooking instructions and fully cook them or, better yet, learn how to properly sprout them. You may benefit from a digestive enzyme as well.

The Good Fats

The fat phobia from the 1980s and '90s persists today, as evidenced by the "low-fat" products still lining grocery store aisles. This drives me bonkers, and it is so wrong. You should always have some fat on your plate. It is incredibly good-mood-promoting!

Take a look at the ingredients label of that low-fat product next time you're at the grocery store. Chances are it's full of sugar or other nasty additives. Fat adds flavor, so when fat is removed, some other ingredient must replace it to boost flavor. That usually means sugar, artificial sweeteners or chemicals you can't pronounce and don't recognize. This is a very unjoyous thing to do to food! Plus, when you remove the fat, you limit the secretion of your satiation hormone, leptin.

Your brain is actually a very fatty organ—it's composed of up to 60 percent fat. The myelin sheaths that cover your nerves and are essential for proper nerve function are literally made of fat—in fact, they are up to 85 percent fat. Fat helps your brain function because it aids in the transmission of nerve impulses. Just as the oil on your bike chain helps you ride faster, fat in your brain helps neural impulses transmit more efficiently. Studies have shown that people who take antidepressants have better results when they supplement with omega-3 fats.

Not all fats are created equal, but to remain healthy, we must eat all kinds of fats, both saturated and unsaturated. Many health experts give a thumbs-down to saturated fat, but this is poor advice. Saturated fat in excess is harmful (as is anything in excess), but our bodies still need it in smaller amounts. It gives your cellular membranes structure and stability. Saturated fat is not very susceptible to damage, and therefore provides excellent protection for your cells.

Since most people eat enough saturated fats but too few omega-3 fats (an unsaturated fat), most of the good fats I recommend below are lower in saturated fat, with the exception of coconut oil. (Read more about the superfood coconut oil on page 94.)

SOURCES OF GOOD FAT

Some of these foods are also a good source of protein.

Fish

- anchovies
- mackerel (not king)
- Pacific cod
- sablefish
- sardines
- wild salmon (limit canned to no more than once every two weeks due to BPA)

Note: Do not eat shark, swordfish, king mackerel or tilefish because they contain high levels of mercury. Limit albacore tuna to 6 oz (170 g) per week.

Nuts and Seeds

- almonds
- cashews
- chia and flaxseeds
- macadamia nuts
- pecans
- walnuts

Oils (Toxins are fat-soluble. As often as possible and when budget allows, be sure to buy organic oils.)

- coconut oil
- extra-virgin olive oil
- flaxseed oil
- hemp oil
- organic butter and ghee (clarified butter)

Dairy Products (in moderation, and only if no food sensitivities are present)

- full-fat organic yogurt
- goat cheese and goat's milk products
- sheep's milk products

D and B-complex Vitamins

Vitamin D is best known for relieving seasonal affective disorder, or SAD, and may help improve mood because it increases levels of serotonin. Our bodies can make plenty of vitamin D from sunshine—this is why it has been appropriately nicknamed the "sunshine vitamin." However, in Canada, our long winters of short days severely limit our exposure to sunshine.

Unfortunately, there is a limited supply of vitamin D in food, but it can be found in salmon, cod, mackerel, sardines, eggs and some dairy products. I recommend vitamin D supplementation. A safe dosage to start with is 1000 IU per day. Speak with your natural healthcare practitioner to find the right dosage for you, as you may need much more than 1000 IU.

B-complex vitamins, especially folate and vitamin B_{12}, are key for a balanced mood because they are involved in the production and metabolism of neurotransmitters that help with mood, especially acetylcholine. Acetylcholine is linked to attention, focus and memory, all of which are affected when you are depressed.

I recommend supplementing with B-complex vitamins, especially if you are on the birth control pill or take medications that may deplete B vitamins. B-complex vitamins work synergistically to support mental health, heart health, energy and metabolism, which is why I recommend taking a B-complex supplement rather than individual B vitamins.

Those on a vegan diet should definitely consider B_{12} supplementation because when you don't eat animal products, it's easy to become deficient. Note that deficiency may not show up on a blood test for years, because B_{12} is stored in your body for up to five years. By the time a deficiency shows up in blood work, you are likely very deficient. Furthermore, it is often said that some plant foods are a source of B_{12}. While this might be true, it's not a type of B_{12} the body can utilize, so supplements are still essential for vegans.

SOURCES OF FOLATE

- black beans
- garbanzo beans
- kidney beans
- leafy greens, such as spinach and collard greens
- lentils
- navy beans
- pinto beans

SOURCES OF VITAMIN B_{12}

- dairy products (in moderation, and only if no food sensitivities are present)
- eggs
- lean beef
- wild salmon

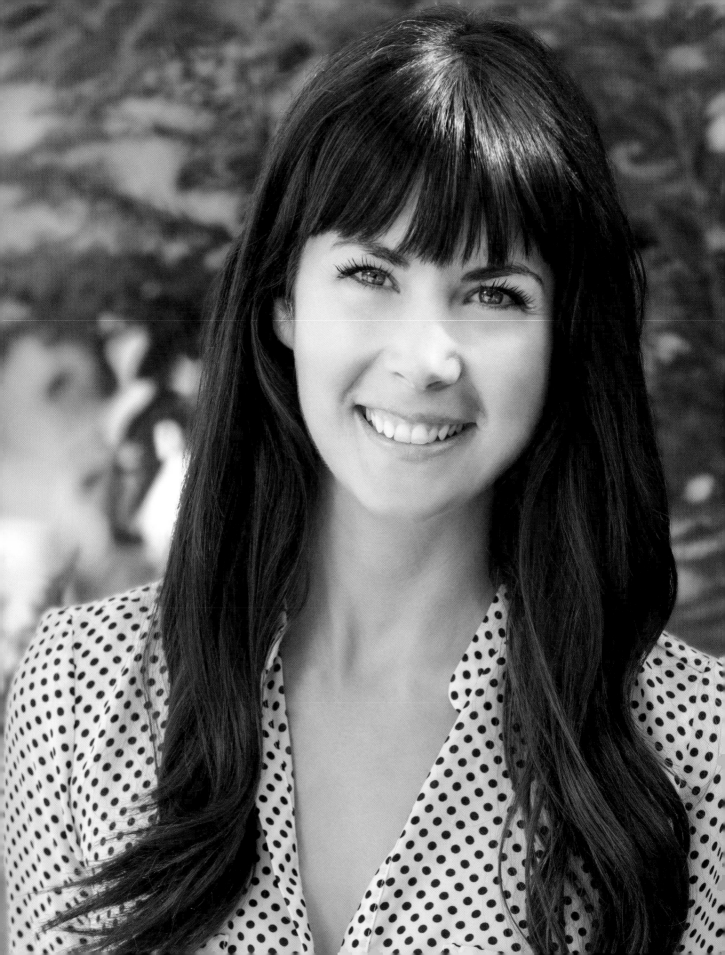

. . .

It's not always about food.
It's also about choosing to
have a joyous attitude.

. . .

5 Joyous Mood Habits

Studies have shown us time and time again that negative thinking may affect our health, lower our immunity, zap our confidence and make us feel very unhappy. The mind and body are intimately connected via the immune, endocrine, central nervous and connective tissue systems. Therefore, there is no disease that isn't simultaneously mental, emotional and physical. Your thoughts create your world, and you create your thoughts. Because of these links, you have an incredible opportunity to take responsibility for your own health and happiness.

The following strategies will help you attain your most joyous healthy self. I highly recommend you choose one or two of these habits and try them out this week.

Strategy 1: Write a Love Letter to Yourself

I once received an email from a woman with the subject line "Desperate: help me get rid of my turkey flap arms." Enough of that! You need to accept and love yourself before you're able to move forward to actually reach your goals and sustain them.

I know it's not that simple, but is it really that complicated? Do you have a choice whether to beat yourself up or not? You sure do! You have power over your own thoughts, and you can choose whether you fill your head with love or with criticism. You have to be your own best cheerleader because there are enough people in the world who may want to criticize you. You've got to stick up for you, especially confronting your own pesky thoughts that do not serve you well.

Here's what to do: whenever a negative thought comes into your head, you are immediately going to replace it with a positive thought. Take out a piece of paper right now and write down three things you love about yourself—a love letter to yourself. For example,

I love my eyes that help me see the beauty in myself.
I love my hips. They make me a gorgeous, curvaceous woman.
I love my arms. They are strong and allow me to embrace others with love.

Keep this piece of paper handy at all times—tape it to your bathroom mirror or put a copy in your wallet. Read it as many times a day as you need to. You will find that eventually you won't need to read it anymore because you will believe it.

Strategy 2: Do a Loving Body Scan

How often do you actually look at yourself naked? How often do you do this without being critical? My guess is rarely or never. I know many women (and men) who won't look at themselves naked in the mirror at all. I used to be one of those women, and I have met many people over the years who felt the same way. When I meet them, I give them all the Loving Body Scan activity. I've done it myself hundreds of times!

I remember the first client I ever recommended this Loving Body Scan to, Karen. I suggested that every morning, before her shower, she stand nude in front of the mirror and look at each part of her body. She stared at me as if I was completely nuts, then started to cry. She told me there was no way she could possibly look at herself naked, because she was afraid of what she might see. I encouraged her to start slowly—that each week she look at one new body part and say loving, positive things about that body part, starting with her feet and moving up to her legs, hips, tummy, breasts, arms and finally her face.

Guess what? Karen followed this advice, and although it took quite a few months to get her to look at her whole self completely naked, she did it! Karen continues to do this Loving Body Scan every so often, especially when she is not feeling her best, and she found it boosted her self-esteem immensely.

Joyous Tip

Love your body! Try looking at yourself completely naked a few times a week. It will be tough at first, but it's a great way to build self-confidence and self-love.

Level 1: After you have a shower, **with your towel on**, go to a full-length mirror and look at yourself for five minutes. While you are looking at yourself, repeat the affirmation below. It may feel silly or embarrassing, but don't worry, no one will hear you. Do this every day for at least one week.

Level 2: When you are ready to graduate to the next level, after you have a shower, **with your towel covering half your body**, look at the lower half of your body in the mirror for five minutes. While you are looking at yourself, repeat the affirmation.

Level 3: Ready for level 3? After you have a shower, **with your towel off**, start by looking at your feet and your legs, then move your way up, looking at your entire body for five minutes in the mirror. While you are looking at yourself, repeat the affirmation.

. . .

"I have a beautiful body. I love all parts of me. I am perfectly perfect."

. . .

Strategy 3: Move That Sexy Booty!

There's no shortage of studies that prove the mood-boosting and serotonin-inducing effects of breaking into a good sweat. Don't forget that exercise also increases levels of the queen bee neurotransmitter, nitric oxide. This translates into an improvement in your mood and self-esteem. Exercise is also an excellent way to help your body better detoxify. When you increase your circulation, you help move waste products out of your cells. Plus you get a rosy-cheeked glow!

Exercise provides you with a full-on megadose of feel-good hormones. It's a great way to feel sexy instantly. In fact, exercise has been shown to be as effective as some antidepressants. A 1999 study published in *The Archives of Internal Medicine* divided a group of 156 men and women suffering from depression into three groups. One group was given the antidepressant Zoloft, the second group took part in an aerobic exercise program, and the third group was given the exercise program *and* the antidepressant. After sixteen weeks, 60 to 70 percent of the participants *in all three groups* were no longer showing symptoms of major depression, suggesting that exercise alone was just as effective in treating depression as were an antidepressant or an antidepressant and exercise combined. Even better, when the scientists checked in with the participants six months later, they found that those who exercised regularly after the study were less likely to have relapsed into depression, regardless of which treatment they received during the original study.

If you already exercise, in your next workout, dial it up a notch. Make it a little more intense by going up a level in weights or add more or faster intervals in your cardio. Perhaps try a completely different activity, such as kickboxing, or join a recreational sports league. Keep lots of variety in your exercise routine so it doesn't lose its effect.

If you don't get regular exercise, start doing something, anything, today. Get up off the couch (or get away from your desk) and go for a ten-minute brisk walk. Each week, add more time to this walk, or perhaps start doing some simple body-weight-bearing exercises at home. Try walking lunges, push-ups or squats.

Strategy 4: Do a Weekly Brain Dump

I took a course called "The Psychology of Disease" that discussed how our emotions are connected to the health of our body. One of the best exercises I learned in this class was a "brain dump" that helps purge any junk thoughts you accumulated during the day before you go to sleep at night.

Here's how you do the brain dump: Write a full page, without lifting your pen from your paper, of all the thoughts—the good, bad and ugly—that are in your mind. When you are done, take this piece of paper and either burn it (safely, please!) or tear it up into tiny shreds and toss it out. This stream-of-consciousness exercise is a very effective way to rid yourself of negative thought patterns that do not serve you well.

Strategy 5: Get Fresh Air on Your Beautiful Face

I know I don't need to convince you of this, because you probably already know how good you feel when you're near water or taking a walk in a park with trees and grass, but science proves this link! A large study from the United Kingdom shows that green space is a powerful mood enhancer and improves self-esteem.

Get outside and get fresh air on your beautiful face every day if you can. Even better, take your entire workout outside. If the weather is not ideal for outdoor exercise, just bundle up! Adding some sweat to the equation by getting your heart rate up (see strategy 3) will make your body feel even more joyous.

10 Emotional Eating Quick Tips

So you've had a crappy day, done your brain dump exercise and still feel like slurping back a whole bottle of wine or a pint of ice cream? Here are some tips to keep you feeling like a superstar. Remember, eating well and living well today will ensure that you wake up tomorrow feeling awesome!

1. Avoid Trigger Foods

Sugary treats, baked goods, chocolate, candies, white rice, white pasta, potato chips and fried foods can all promote blood sugar imbalances (which can put you in a bad mood) or put you into a food coma that makes you feel like crap the next day. This is a vicious cycle, because the next day you are likely going to feel guilty (but please try not to, because "food guilt" won't get you anywhere). It's even possible your digestion will feel off and possibly trigger you to do the same thing again the next evening. You can stop this cycle by cutting out these trigger foods for two weeks and evaluating how amazing you feel. Many of the recipes in this book will make you feel fabulous.

2. Tame Your Stress

Alternate nostril breathing, also known as *nadi shodhana*, is a simple but powerful relaxation exercise I learned in yoga class from Michelle Uy, my favorite yoga teacher and the co-founder of Eat Well Feel Well. It's a great way to calm your mind and nervous system, and if you're feeling tired, it's a great energy booster. The left side of your brain is associated with thinking and the right side with feeling. Alternate nostril breathing helps restore any imbalances in the brain so that you can access your whole brain—plus reduce stress.

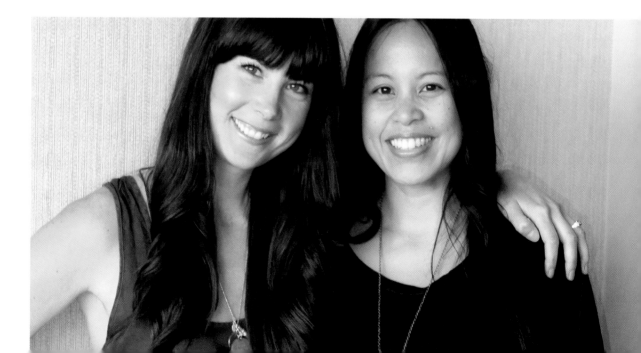

1. Sit in a comfortable position with a straight back. You want to feel as though you have a long spine.

2. Rest your left hand on your lap. Bring your right thumb to your right nostril and your fourth finger to your left nostril. Your index and your middle finger will rest at the top of your nose.

3. Take a deep breath in through both nostrils. As you exhale, plug your right nostril with your thumb and exhale through your left nostril.

4. Keeping your right nostril plugged, take a deep breath in through the left nostril, plug your left nostril with your fourth finger and exhale through the right nostril.

5. Inhale through the right nostril, plug the right nostril with your thumb and exhale through the left nostril.

6. Inhale through the left nostril, plug the left nostril with your fourth finger and exhale through the right nostril.

7. Continue for a few more rounds.

8. You can start off doing this for three minutes and gradually work your way up to ten minutes.

9. Sit quietly for a few moments after you are done.

Yoga, meditation or relaxation exercises, such as breathing deeply with your hand on your belly at night before bed to ensure you are taking deep, delicious breaths, will calm your nervous system and help you better manage stress. Alternatively, take a warm bath with essential oils like lavender or drink relaxing teas like chamomile or passionflower before bed.

3. Have a Hunger Reality Check

Next time you want to eat something, ask yourself, Am I hungry physically or emotionally? Give the craving a little time to pass. Being in the present moment and creating awareness around feelings of hunger and appetite help you better assess whether you want to eat out of boredom or to relieve negative feelings, or because you are actually hungry.

Thirsty or hungry? Did you know that thirst is often confused with hunger? Stay well hydrated and drink at least one or two glasses of pure water at least an hour before each meal (by a glass I mean 1 to 2 cups/250 to 500 mL). Not only will this prevent you from overeating, but if it's not actually time for your body to eat, this will prevent you from eating when you are in fact just thirsty, since thirst and hunger often get confused.

4. Keep a Food Diary

You've heard me say this before but that's just because it's such an effective strategy. Write down when you eat, what you eat and how you're feeling when you eat it. This will help reveal the connections between your mood and food. Remember that there's a food and wellness journal at the back of this book.

5. Get Support

Often we eat for reasons other than hunger. Getting support by sharing your feelings with others is a much better way to address your emotions than diving into a bag of potato chips. The key is to do something enjoyable that doesn't involve food: call a friend, meet a friend for tea, join a book club, take up a hobby or join a recreational sports league.

6. Do Something That Makes You Feel Good

Science tells us that we gravitate toward foods that conjure happy memories because they may release brain chemicals such as dopamine, the feel-good hormone. If mac and cheese was your feel-good food as a kid, it may very well be your go-to meal when you've had a rough day, as it stimulates the pleasure center of your brain. Instead of eating that mac and cheese, do something that makes you feel good. Exercise is one of the best feel-good activities that you never regret doing once you are done. Take your dog for a brisk walk, ride your bike, go for a light jog, get out in nature and go for a hike.

7. Take Away Temptation

As the old saying goes, Out of sight, out of mind. Don't keep a stock of unhealthy comfort foods like potato chips, ice cream or candy in your home if they're hard for you to resist. Try out the healthy recipes in this book instead!

8. Don't Deprive Yourself

I hear this often from my clients: you eat "clean" all week, and then the weekend comes and you feel like a cookie monster—or worse, you want to eat everything fatty, sugary and unhealthy. What's happening here? Deprivation can actually increase your food cravings and appetite hormones. Let yourself enjoy an occasional treat. Above all, eat food that tastes good all the time—healthy can and should be delicious. You can make healthy swaps that taste just as delicious as their unhealthy counterparts (see page 126 for a list of healthy substitutions). For example, when you feel like eating chocolate brownie ice cream, why not try my Chocolate Mint Pudding on page 270 or the Chili and Cinnamon Chocolate Bark on page 264. These recipes are truly guilt-free indulgences.

9. Snack Healthy

There are plenty of easy, tasty and healthy snack options out there! Almonds and dried cranberries; a sliced apple with 2 tbsp (30 mL) of nut butter or 5 walnuts; veggies with 2 tbsp (30 mL) of hummus; or the Overnight Strawberry Chia Pudding on page 157 are all well-balanced snacks that will keep your belly quiet and your taste buds joyous.

10. Get Enough Sleep

Studies prove that sleep-deprived people eat more carbs, sugars and unhealthy foods. When you get less than six hours of sleep, your appetite-stimulating hormone, ghrelin, is increased and your satiation-signaling hormone, leptin, is decreased—talk about a double whammy! Get to bed by 10:30 or 11 every night and aim to get seven and a half to nine hours of uninterrupted sleep each night in complete darkness.

Joyous Tip

Go dark. Sleeping in complete darkness allows your body to get into a deep phase of sleep and release melatonin, your sleep hormone. This hormone is released by the pineal gland, a walnut-sized gland in your brain. The pineal gland senses light and darkness, so a dark room is critical to a good night's sleep. Get yourself an eye mask or blackout curtains if need be and get your beauty sleep!

Green Pea and Sun-Dried Tomato Dip (or Pesto)

Michelle Uy, a yoga instructor and co-founder of Eat Well Feel Well, has made this recipe several times for potlucks I've attended, and it's full of flavor. She also loves making it just for herself after a long day of teaching. The perfect comfort food. Michelle says, "I love this dish because it's versatile and so simple to make. Choose your favorite pasta to accompany the pesto, or as a dip, serve it with crackers or spread it on celery sticks. Happy eating!"

Makes 3 to 4 cups (750 mL to 1 L) of dip or 3 to 4 servings of pesto

D Detox **V** Vegan **DF** Dairy-free **GF** Gluten-free **J** Joyous Comfort

2 cups (500 mL) fresh or thawed frozen green peas

1 cup (250 mL) drained oil-packed sun-dried tomatoes

½ cup (125 mL) walnuts

1 tbsp (15 mL) lemon juice

3 cloves garlic

¼ cup (60 mL) olive oil

Sea salt and pepper

½ cup (125 mL) grated Parmesan cheese
   (or nutritional yeast for a non-dairy option)

If making pesto:
¼ cup (60 mL) water
¼ cup (60 mL) chopped fresh basil and/or parsley

In a food processor, combine green peas, sun-dried tomatoes, walnuts, lemon juice and garlic. Pulse several times. With motor running, drizzle in olive oil until mixture is smooth.
If making pesto: drizzle in water to thin out the pesto.

Transfer to a bowl and season with salt and pepper. Stir in Parmesan cheese.
If making pesto: sprinkle with basil and/or parsley just before serving.

4
JOYOUS
DETOX
SOLUTIONS

When you take a break from certain foods—or rather, the food-like substances I'll talk about in this chapter—and instead eat the foods and recipes recommended here and in the Joyous Health 10-Day Meal Plan in chapter 6, you will feel renewed and completely rejuvenated.

An amazing sense of empowerment comes from taking a break from foods that don't serve you well. Think of every morsel you eat as energy that literally becomes part of your body. Your body creates your cells from the food you eat, so when you eat vibrant foods, such as fruits, vegetables, healthy fats and high-quality proteins, you will feel amazing, and this feeling will be reflected outwardly. Remember, outside beauty is merely a reflection of the inside health of your body.

When my clients stop eating processed foods and focus on whole foods with natural detoxifying compounds, they experience some (or all) of these benefits:

- improved energy
- no more brain fog
- bright, glowing skin
- whiter whites of eyes
- weight loss
- better digestion and elimination
- improved sleep and libido (*ooh la la!*)
- a sense of peace and joy

Why You Should Detox

Over the past seventy-five years, more than a hundred thousand chemicals have been developed across every industry. Whether the purpose of these chemicals is to speed the growth of crops or to ease soap-scum removal on your bathtub, the large majority of these chemicals are not doing the health of our bodies or the planet any good. Check out these alarming statistics.

- Of the 2.5 million tons of pesticides used each year worldwide, less than 0.1 percent actually make it to the pest. The rest remain in our food and environment.
- Since 1945, pesticide use has increased 3300 percent.
- Environmental toxins have been found in the breast milk of over 90 percent of women studied in North America.
- High levels of environmental toxins have been found in the fat tissue and urine of over 80 percent of North American adults.

But I have joyous news! Despite what you may have heard, to detoxify, you don't need to starve yourself while sweating naked on a rock in the desert for ten days! I'll show you some simple, natural and very effective steps you can take to help your body better detoxify itself.

Foods to Eliminate from Your Diet

The first step in detoxifying your body is to stop consuming the following foods for at least two weeks. That's about the amount of time it will take for you to notice a difference in your body. Use the food and wellness journal at the back of this book to evaluate how you feel each day.

Ditch the Cow's Milk

The sterile, white pasteurized and homogenized milk for sale in grocery stores is nothing like the raw milk our great-grandparents were drinking years ago. (In Canada, raw, or unpasteurized, milk has not been legal for sale to consumers since 1991. In slightly more than half the US states, the sale of raw milk is not prohibited, but it's not always easy to get.) Pasteurization and homogenization are the main reasons why cow's milk is hard to digest and mucus-forming. A protein in cow's milk called casein also contributes to the dairy-digestion issues that many people experience. Intolerance to dairy and dairy products is one of the most common food sensitivities today.

WHAT IS PASTEURIZATION? Pasteurization is the process of heating a food, in this case milk, to a high temperature to destroy all the bacteria in it—the good *and* the bad— essentially rendering the milk sterile. However, good bacteria are essential for a healthy immune and digestive system.

WHAT IS HOMOGENIZATION? Homogenization is a process that changes the molecular structure of the fat globules in milk so they stay integrated in the milk instead of separating as cream. Before the days of homogenization, that layer of fat could be spooned off the top, and the milk was easier for fat-digesting enzymes to break down.

Both processes change the chemical makeup of the milk, making it harder to digest and more likely to cause allergies and food intolerances. And we cannot ignore the fact that many people, when they are weaned, stop producing the enzyme lactase, which is needed to break down milk sugar, called lactose.

So why are so many people still slurping their latte from the coffee shop or pouring milk on their morning cereal? Good question! Probably because they are not aware of the problems the cow's milk is causing them, problems such as gas and bloating, constipation and diarrhea, acne and allergic responses such as a runny nose, asthma, skin rashes and irritability. These are some of the most common milk-related problems I see with my clients. The best side effect I've noticed when my clients ditch cow's milk is that they say bye-bye to face puffiness caused by inflammation.

You can still enjoy a latte or a milk-like liquid on your morning granola with these equally delicious alternatives to cow's milk:

- almond milk (see recipe on page 170)
- brown rice milk
- coconut milk (see recipe on page 168)
- goat's milk
- hemp milk (see recipe on page 170)
- oat milk
- quinoa milk

If you drink goat's milk, do so in moderation, because it can cause some of the same problems that cow's milk does, although there is less of the problematic casein protein in goat's milk, making it easier to digest.

Worried about losing the calcium if you say goodbye to cow's milk? Eat (or drink) more of these calcium-rich foods:

- almonds
- collard greens, kale, spinach and turnip greens
- goat's milk
- molasses
- navy beans
- salmon and sardines
- sesame seeds and tahini (sesame paste)
- tempeh (fermented tofu)—choose organic whenever possible

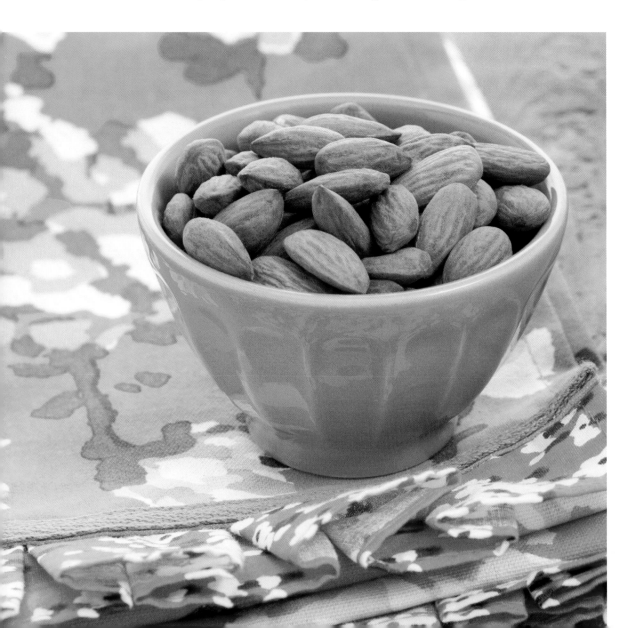

Ditch the Wheat

According to naturopath Dr. Carolee Bateson-Koch, the author of *Allergies: Disease in Disguise*, when you repeatedly consume a specific food, you deplete your enzyme systems, which can lead to a sensitivity to that food. For example, if you eat a white-flour bagel every day, you are much more likely to become sensitive to white flour because your body becomes deficient in the very enzymes needed to break down that flour. (And let's not forget that today's wheat, just like cow's milk, is not the same as what our great-grandparents were eating. Most of it is now genetically modified.)

North Americans eat far too much wheat, as evidenced by the number of people who have become intolerant to it. As new clients begin to work with me, I see in their food journals, time and again, that almost every day they eat white or whole-wheat toast for breakfast, some sort of sandwich or wrap at lunch and pasta or bread with dinner. That's a one-way ticket to becoming sensitive to wheat! Symptoms of sensitivity to wheat are vast and varied and include itchy skin, eczema, digestive problems, fatigue and depression.

Dr. William Davis, author of *Wheat Belly*, says that wheat should be eliminated from our diet. "Because of wheat's incredible capacity to send blood sugar levels straight up, initiate the glucose-insulin roller coaster ride that drives appetite, generate addictive brain-active exorphins, and grow visceral fat, it is the one essential food to eliminate in a serious effort to prevent, reduce, or eliminate diabetes."

If you are going to eat wheat, make sure it's certified organic and choose "sprouted" wheat instead. When wheat is sprouted, it is far easier to digest and higher in protein (which helps to reduce blood sugar). You will find sprouted wheat breads in the health food store. One of my favorite brands is Silver Hills Bakery.

Want to take it one step further? You may want to consider eliminating gluten. Gluten is the protein in barley, oats, rye, spelt, wheat and kamut, as well as all flours and foods made with these grains. Taking a break from gluten will help you assess whether you may be intolerant to it. If you ordinarily experience symptoms of food sensitivity and they vanish or are significantly reduced when you stop consuming gluten, then you have your answer! Be sure to check out the recipes in this book that are free of gluten, noted by a GF symbol.

Ditch the Refined Sugar

This evil white stuff has many negative health implications, including lowering immune system function, promoting type 2 diabetes and making us fat. North Americans are eating far too much sugar. In fact, some experts believe the average person eats 150 pounds of sugar every year!

Most people know that eating candy and pastries every day doesn't exactly promote good health. However, sugar is hidden in food items that you may think are good for you. Read the labels on your pasta sauces, salad dressings, cereals, granola bars, energy bars, flavored yogurts, low-fat products and snack foods. These are where refined sugars are usually hidden. You might be shocked to discover that your favorite flavored yogurt contains as much sugar as ice cream.

Here's what to look for when checking a list of ingredients for hidden refined sugars: brown sugar, raw sugar, cane sugar, mannitol, sorbitol and just about anything ending in "ose": sucrose, glucose, fructose, lactose, maltose and dextrose. Avoid high-fructose corn syrup at all costs—I'll tell you why in a bit. Chapter 6 will guide you to healthy sugar substitutes.

The bottom line is that you should save treats for a treat and truly enjoy every morsel when you have them. If you want to indulge in that chocolate almond croissant, then make sure you really enjoy it and don't do it every day.

Ditch the Processed Soy Products

Many vegans and vegetarians use soy products as a staple in their diet because soy is an excellent source of protein and calcium. However, I do not recommend processed soy, including soy burgers, soy cheese, soy yogurt, soy milk, soy hot dogs, soy flour, tofu, soy protein or soy formula. They are the junk foods of the soy industry.

Here are just a few of the problems associated with soy:

- Most "natural" soy products are bathed in a toxic chemical solvent known as hexane.

- Soy is a very common food allergen that often results in inflammation.

- Unfermented soy (e.g., tofu) contains enzyme inhibitors and is therefore extremely hard to digest.

- Research has found that the high levels of phytic acid found in soy reduce the assimilation of calcium, magnesium, copper, iron and zinc. The phytic acid can be neutralized by preparation methods such as soaking, sprouting and long, slow cooking.

- Research on the phytoestrogens in soy and their effect on the body is inconclusive and often conflicting. In my own practice, many of my clients find it extremely beneficial to remove soy from their diet, and some even find it lessens the severity of PMS.

If you wish to eat soy products, do so only if you have no sensitivity to them, and eat only fermented soy, such as tempeh, miso, natto and tamari. Try my flavorful Amy's Tempeh Chili recipe on page 239.

Other Foods to Ditch

Take a break for two weeks from these other foods for your most joyous health:

- alcoholic beverages
- corn
- fast food, including fried foods (fries, onion rings, chicken fingers) and all junk foods (potato chips)
- frozen dinners (usually full of salt and other food additives)
- peanuts
- the three white nasties: white rice, white pasta and white bread

Unjoyous Food Additives

Stick to this general rule when buying foods in a package: make sure all the ingredients are ones you recognize as food, and remember that *less is more*. In other words, the fewer the ingredients, the better the food is for you. A bag of apples doesn't have an ingredients list or flashy packaging yelling health claims, does it? Of course not. Healthy food doesn't need a claim. On the other hand, food that's trying to hide something is usually plastered with deceptive marketing claims such as "low-fat," "cholesterol-free" or "trans-fat free."

When grocery shopping, always read the ingredients list on a package and avoid artificial colors, flavors, preservatives and sweeteners. That word says it all! *Artificial* ingredients have no place or purpose in the human body. Some have been shown to promote tumor growth in rats. How do you avoid them? Read your labels.

Artificial Colors

Petroleum-based coloring agents are used to give a more pleasant color to, or mask an unappealing color in, foods such as desserts and sweets, snack foods, mac and cheese, condiments and spreads, and beverages such as pop and fruit juice. You will also find them in cosmetics and personal care products. Most artificial food colors are known carcinogens and allergens.

In the United States, Food, Drug and Cosmetic (FD&C) numbers are assigned to artificial colors, making it easy to spot them in ingredients lists. In Canada, manufacturers are required only to use the term "color" in their labeling, making no distinction between artificial and (usually safe) natural colors.

Joyous Tip

Use your eagle eye with food labels. When grocery shopping and reading ingredients labels, ask yourself, "Will this ingredient lead me toward more joyous health?" If you easily answer no, then put the package back on the shelf.

Artificial Flavors

Approximately two thousand chemicals make up the various flavor enhancers in our food supply. Food manufacturers are not required to list each individual synthetic flavoring (the formulas are considered "trade secrets"), so "artificial flavor" on the ingredients label can encompass a long list of mystery chemicals. One of the most common flavor enhancers is monosodium glutamate, otherwise known as MSG. It is commonly found in Chinese food, potato chips, soups, sauces, gravy mixes, water-packed tuna and dry-roasted nuts. MSG can trigger asthma and cause headaches, digestive problems and chest pains. In 1978, it was banned from baby food because it was shown to cause damage to the brain stem in infants. If you buy only real food that doesn't come in a package, it's quite easy to avoid flavorings such as MSG.

Joyous Tip

MSG has many other names. Watch out for hydrolyzed vegetable protein, autolyzed yeast, hydrolyzed yeast, vegetable powder or natural flavor. Yes, you read that right, *natural* flavor! If you do happen to ingest MSG, you'll need vitamin B_6 to metabolize it. Therefore, supplementing with B_6 could help stop reactions to MSG. But a much better option is to avoid products with MSG altogether.

Artificial Preservatives

Preservatives give foods a longer shelf life. Salt, vinegar and honey are natural preservatives, but synthetically produced ones do nothing for the health of your body. Two such artificial preservatives, BHA and BHT, are commonly found in cereals, frozen dinners, baked goods, fruit juices and chewing gum. They were actually banned from children's cereals in Canada (and banned completely in England) because they can affect the nervous system and cause behavioral problems in children. However, these preservatives are still added to many foods. Studies have shown that BHT and BHA inhibit growth, cause weight loss and damage the liver, kidneys and testicles in rats.

Sulfites are often added to foods to prevent them from turning brown. They come in many forms, including sodium bisulfate, sodium sulfite and potassium sulfite. People with asthma and those who already suffer from allergies are especially sensitive to sulfites. The most common products containing artificial sulfites are wine, dried fruits, potato chips, frozen fries, fruit snacks and frozen dinners.

Nitrates and nitrites are added to cured meats and meat products to prevent browning. Have you ever wondered why bacon or hot dogs look so pink? That's thanks to preservatives such as nitrates and nitrites. The problem is that nitrates and nitrites react with secondary amines found in protein-containing foods to form what are called nitrosamines, and nitrosamines have been found to cause cancer in animals. Dr. William Lijinsky, of the National Cancer Institute, considers nitrites in meat to be the most dangerous food additive today and a major contributor to the development of cancer. Although more recent research indicates they are less harmful than previously thought, I still recommend avoiding them.

. . . .

Joyous Tip

"Natural" luncheon meats? If you see the ingredient "celery root extract" listed, steer clear! It's the same thing as sodium nitrate, which converts to sodium nitrite when eaten.

. . . .

Artificial Sweeteners

The four big artificial sweeteners lurking in our food supply are aspartame (NutraSweet and Equal), acesulfame potassium (Sunnette and Sweet One), sucralose (Splenda) and saccharin (Sweet'N Low). They can be found in gum, flavored and low-fat yogurts, jam, protein powders, energy bars and cereals, and toothpaste. In the United States, 75 percent of adverse reactions to food additives are caused by aspartame, according to the Food and Drug Administration, yet it remains on the market.

Fifty percent of aspartame is the amino acid phenylalanine. Too much phenylalanine is a neurotoxin; it excites the neurons in the brain to the point of cellular death. In fact, ADD/ADHD and emotional and behavioral disorders can be triggered by too much phenylalanine in the diet. Read your labels and avoid artificial sweeteners. See page 122 for a list of the many healthy natural sweeteners, including honey and applesauce, that you can use instead.

Top 7 Foods to Avoid

Here are the foods I recommend you avoid beyond what we've already talked about.

Microwaved Foods

Use your microwave as an extra cupboard, because it doesn't do your food any good! A study published in the *Journal of the Science of Food and Agriculture* found that broccoli cooked in a microwave oven lost up to 97 percent of its nutrients. Cooking of any kind can result in nutrient loss, but sautéing will cause much less, especially if very little water is used. If you must defrost something, avoid plastic or plastic wrap in the microwave, as plastic molecules can leach into food.

Microwaved popcorn is a definite no-no. The lining of the microwave bag is coated with a substance that when heated produces perfluorooctanoic acid, or PFOA, thought to be a carcinogen. And it gets worse. You may have heard of "miner's lung," but have you ever heard of "popcorn worker's lung"? It's a respiratory disease reported in people who work in the factories where this food-like substance is created. It's caused by inhaling another dangerous chemical, diacetyl, which is used to make the fake butter flavoring.

Margarine

As Michael Pollan states in his book *In Defense of Food*, if a prepared food can last days to weeks on end, it's not real food. Just say no to margarine! Sure, it comes from vegetables that are rich in omega-6 fats, but we get too many of these fats as it is. Plus, those omega-6 fats must go through a whole series of processes to become margarine. It is a completely chemically altered food. Avoid it!

High-Fructose Corn Syrup

High-fructose corn syrup, or HFCS, is corn syrup that's been chemically modified to have more fructose than glucose. Because fructose is sweeter than glucose, food manufacturers don't need to use as much of it to make a food sweeter, saving them a ton of money. The problem is, HFCS overloads the liver with fructose, and the liver converts that to glucose, and this excess glucose converts to fat. HFCS is strongly implicated in the rapid rise of obesity and type 2 diabetes. It may also increase inflammation, which puts you at a greater risk for heart disease. Read your labels, because it's found in many breads, baked goods, processed foods, flavored yogurts, dressings and sauces, and cough syrups. In Canada it is also called glucose/fructose.

Canned Foods

Although I do have a few recipes in this book that call for canned beans, the brands I recommend do not contain bisphenol A, or BPA. If you must buy a canned product, look for a brand labeled "BPA-free." BPA is an estrogen mimicker and can cause hormonal imbalances (see page 77). It was once declared a toxic substance in Canada, and even though that designation was later removed, I still recommend you avoid it. The Environmental Working Group estimates that up to 90 percent of canned foods contain BPA.

I know that canned soup can be über-convenient, but fresh is far tastier and healthier. In fact, a study from the Harvard School of Public Health found that people who consumed a serving of canned soup each day for five days had more than a 1000 percent increase in urinary BPA concentrations compared with those who consumed fresh soup daily for five days. Try Mama Bea's Curry Lentil Soup on page 188 and go fresh!

Fruit-Flavored Fat-Free Yogurt

There is a big misconception that low-fat fruit-flavored yogurt is a healthy product. First of all, don't be afraid of fat! As you learned earlier, fat is essential for satiation. Most of these fruit-flavored yogurts, though, are full of sugar or artificial sweeteners. Buy plain yogurt and add your own flavorings, such as cinnamon, fresh fruit or raw honey. Even better, try kefir, which is a fermented yogurt product very high in good bacteria. There is coconut and water kefir as well, perfect if you're dairy-intolerant. Furthermore, try to choose organic when consuming any dairy products.

Fruit Juice and Pop

Fruit juices contain very little nutrition (unless they are fortified with synthetic vitamins, which I do not recommend), and juice rapidly spikes blood sugar. Plus, wouldn't you rather eat your calories than drink them? As for pop, there is absolutely nothing in it of any value to the human body—although you will certainly get a nice dose of the very food additives I suggest you avoid, from artificial coloring to artificial flavoring, as well as a megawatt amount of inorganic phosphorus, of which your body absorbs nearly 100 percent. Excess phosphorus can steal calcium from bones and teeth. And of course, you already know that sugar or artificial sweeteners are definite no-nos. If you want juice, make it yourself. There are some delicious recipes on page 174.

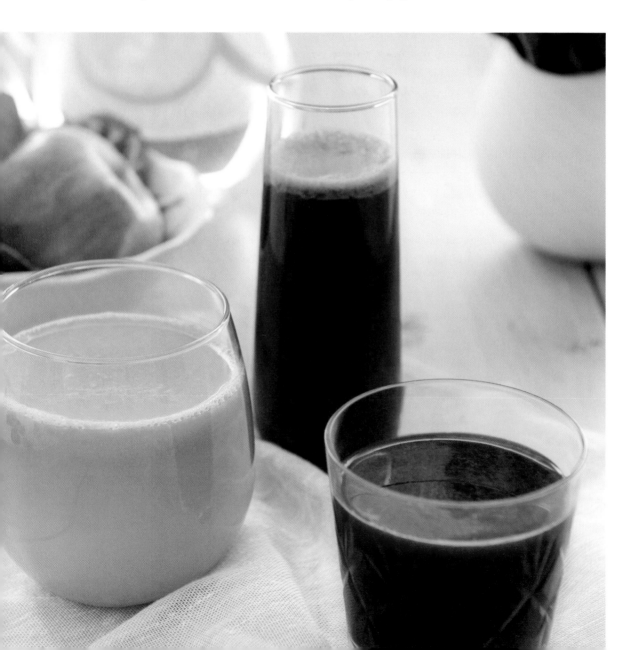

JOYOUS WARNING

What is BPA? Bisphenol A is an industrial chemical that has been banned for use in baby bottles in Canada but is still found in many plastic products. It is used to make these two synthetic products:

- Polycarbonate: a clear, rigid, shatter-resistant plastic found in a wide variety of consumer products, including food and drink containers.

- Epoxy resins: used in industrial adhesives and high-performance coatings. Epoxy coatings line most of the 131 billion food cans (especially tomato and soup) and beverage cans (especially coconut milk) made annually in the United States, according to the Environmental Working Group.

PROBLEMS WITH BPA: BPA is a synthetic estrogen that, even in the smallest amounts, can disrupt the delicate endocrine system. It has been linked to infertility, breast and reproductive system cancers, obesity, type 2 diabetes, early puberty and behavioral changes in children. A 2010 Statistics Canada survey found that 91 percent of Canadians have BPA in their bodies.

GOOD NEWS: A study done by Environmental Health Perspectives found that families that ate fresh food for three days, with no canned food, and using only glass storage containers, experienced a 60 percent reduction of BPA in their urine. Taking a break from canned food will reduce your body's accumulation of this hormone-disrupting chemical.

Because of the acidic nature of tomatoes, any canned product will contain low levels of BPA. To reduce your exposure, purchase tomatoes in a glass bottle. Eden Organic is a great brand for both tomatoes and canned beans. The canned beans by Eden Organic are BPA-free.

Breakfast Cereals and Cereal Bars

This is food marketing at its finest—advertising products as "healthy" when they are full of sugar and refined grains that have been stripped of B vitamins, essential fatty acids and minerals. These products also contain additives such as flavorings, colorings and preservatives. Of course there are some healthy exceptions, so you just need to be a food detective and read your labels carefully. Also, don't be afraid to contact a food manufacturer and ask questions about ingredients you don't recognize.

BEST NATURAL DETOXIFIERS

- artichokes
- beets and beet greens
- berries, including goji berries, blueberries, strawberries, raspberries and blackberries
- cruciferous vegetables, including broccoli, Brussels sprouts, cauliflower and cabbage
- fennel
- fermented foods such as sauerkraut, kefir and kombucha
- fresh fruits such as apples, pears, lemons and avocados
- fresh herbs, including parsley, cilantro, basil, rosemary and oregano
- garlic
- ginger root
- green tea
- leafy greens, including kale, arugula, Swiss chard, collard greens, spinach, bok choy and dandelion greens
- nuts and seeds, especially Brazil nuts, pumpkin seeds, chia seeds, flaxseeds, sesame seeds and sunflower seeds (avoid peanuts)
- onions, leeks and chives
- seaweed
- South Asian spices, including turmeric, cloves and cinnamon
- sprouted foods: broccoli sprouts, sprouted lentils, beans and peas

Be sure to check the "Dirty Dozen" list on page 105 and buy organic versions of those foods to reduce your pesticide exposure.

Detox Your Skin with Dry Skin Brushing

Our skin is the largest organ in our body and one of our channels of elimination—toxins leave our body when we sweat. Piling on cosmetics, lotions and potions clogs pores and traps the junk inside.

Dry skin brushing allows the skin to breathe better by unclogging the pores and stimulating the lymphatic system to better eliminate toxins. The lymphatic system is a network of vessels that holds more fluid than you have blood in your body. This network of lymphatic vessels is constantly exchanging nutrients with the blood and picking up waste products for elimination. The lymphatic system doesn't have a pump like the heart, and dry skin brushing helps to move the lymph fluid around. Dry skin brushing is particularly beneficial for stimulating lymphatic drainage from the breasts. Because many toxins are fat soluble, your breasts are fatty organs that can store toxic wastes.

Dry skin brushing is seriously invigorating and beautifying. When you aid the body, especially the skin, to more effectively release toxins, you will glow. Some experts believe that dry skin brushing also helps to eliminate cellulite—bonus!

DRY SKIN BRUSHING HOW-TO

When: Dry skin brushing should be done three to four times a week on dry skin before showering or bathing.

What: Use a natural-fiber brush with a wood or bamboo handle. The bristles should be comfortably uncomfortable. That is, they should stimulate but not scratch the skin. Test the brush out on your arm at the health food store.

How: Apply just enough pressure that the brush feels stimulating or "tingly." It should not hurt. You may see "chalky" white marks on your skin for a short time after brushing. This is normal.

Where: Start with the bottom of your feet and work up your body, moving the brush in a circular motion toward your heart. Make sure you spend more time where you have lymph nodes, such as the back of your knees, inside the elbows and your armpits. When you reach your breasts, brush toward your armpits and around your nipples to stimulate lymphatic drainage.

. . . .

Joyous Tip

What not to brush: Avoid brushing your nipples. They are too sensitive for a dry skin brush. You also shouldn't dry brush your face, unless you have a special brush that has much softer bristles, because the skin on your face is thinner and more sensitive than on the rest of the body.

. . . .

Be a Clean Beauty

According to the Environmental Working Group, studies have found evidence of toxins from personal care products in the blood and urine of babies, teens and adults—yikes! Specific cosmetic ingredients found in our bodies include phthalate plasticizers, paraben preservatives, the pesticide triclosan, synthetic musks and sunscreens. Many studies have shown that these chemicals are hormone disruptors. With prolonged use of various products, they may build up in your body and will disrupt hormones.

How do these toxins end up in our bodies? Quite easily, actually, because what you breathe in from a spray or powder, swallow from a lipstick or gloss, or absorb through your skin from a sunscreen or cosmetic literally gets into you. In fact, it's a more direct route to your bloodstream than actually ingesting something.

Over the years I've seen countless women go clean with their beauty products and have symptoms such as PMS and acne drastically improve. You may think this sounds too good to be true, but it's a fact. I personally have benefited immensely, and now all my personal care products, from shampoo to lipstick, are as natural as possible. If you've never thought about this aspect of your health, now is the time, because the cosmetics industry isn't cleaning up the junk in their products any time soon.

Fortunately, the David Suzuki Foundation has created a list of the top twelve ingredients, known as the "dirty dozen" chemicals, to avoid in personal care products so you can be a clean beauty! Photocopy this guide and carry it with you to ensure none of these ingredients are in the products you buy.

Joyous Tip

Even though it's not required that all ingredients be listed, a product that includes a third-party label such as EcoLogo or Green Seal provides some assurance that the product is safe to use.

Sustainable Shopper's Guide to a Dirty Dozen Ingredients to Avoid in Your Cosmetics

BHA and BHT: In moisturizer, makeup, etc. May cause cancer and interfere with hormone function. Harmful to fish and other wildlife.

Parabens: Widely used in makeup, moisturizers, etc. May interfere with hormone function. Associated with breast cancer.

Coal tar dyes: Look for P-PHENYLENEDIAMINE in hair dyes, and colors identified as "C.I." followed by five digits in other products. Potential to cause cancer and can be contaminated with heavy metals toxic to the brain.

PARFUM: Widely used even in some products marketed as "unscented" (often the last ingredient). Mixture of chemicals that can trigger allergies and asthma. Some linked to cancer and neurotoxicity. Some harmful to fish and other wildlife.

CYCLOMETHICONE and siloxanes: Widely used in moisturizer, makeup, hair products, etc. May interfere with hormone function and damage the liver. Harmful to fish and other wildlife.

PEG: Widely used in conditioners, moisturizers, deodorants, etc. Can be contaminated with 1,4-dioxane, which may cause cancer.

DEA, MEA and TEA: In creamy and foaming products such as moisturizer, shampoo. Can react to form cancer-causing nitrosamines. Harmful to fish and other wildlife.

PETROLATUM: In hair products, lip balm/lipstick, skin care products. Petroleum product that can be contaminated with cancer-causing impurities.

DIBUTYL PHTHALATE: In nail products. Toxic to reproduction and may interfere with hormone function. Harmful to fish and other wildlife.

SODIUM LAURETH SULFATE (SLES) and SODIUM LAURYL SULFATE (SLS): In products that foam such as shampoo, cleansers, bubble bath. SLES can be contaminated with 1,4-dioxane, which may cause cancer. SLS may damage liver. Harmful to fish and other wildlife.

Formaldehyde-releasing preservatives: Look for DMDM Hydantoin, Diazolidinyl urea, Imidazolidinyl urea, Methenamine, or Quarternium-15. Widely used in hair products, moisturizers, etc. Formaldehyde causes cancer.

TRICLOSAN: In "anti-bacterial" products such as toothpaste, soaps, hand sanitizers. May interfere with hormone function and contribute to antibiotic-resistant bacteria. Harmful to fish and other wildlife.

Source: David Suzuki Foundation, www.DavidSuzuki.org.

You can also find a comprehensive list of more than eighty thousand cosmetic brands on the Environmental Working Group's Skin Deep cosmetics database, which rates products and ingredients for safety. www.ewg.org/skindeep.

Social Detoxing: Edit Your Social Circle

Say what? Yes, do a social detox by editing your social circle! You will be absolutely amazed at how good it feels to do this exercise.

I was introduced to this exercise at a professional development course led by an inspiring professional speaker named Stuart Knight. In a class about relationships, Stuart had us all draw three columns on a sheet of paper and give them the headings "Neutral," "Dump" and "Promote." Let me break the exercise down for you.

Neutral: These are all the relationships you feel neither here nor there about. Meaning they don't add anything particularly wonderful to your life, but they don't bring you down either. Write down the names of everyone you know who falls into this category.

Dump: This is the toughest part. Write down the names of people who bring negativity to your life, perhaps those people who are always in a bad mood, can never sort themselves out or are just bad energy. Of course we all go through ups and downs, and this doesn't mean you dump your longtime girlfriend who's been in a tough situation with her boyfriend for the last couple of months. It's important to be supportive of others going through tough times. But if that girlfriend has been in a constant state of unhappiness for the last two years and all she does is complain and bring nothing joyous to your life whatsoever, perhaps it's time to consider whether this relationship is bringing anything good to your life.

Promote: Write down the names of all the people who challenge and inspire you, people whom you admire and vice versa. These people bring out the best in you, and you feel uplifted and joyous just by being in their presence. These are good people to surround yourself with every day.

Here's what you do next.

Neutral: Either move them into the "dump" category or promote them.

Dump: Don't worry, you don't necessarily need to write a letter or have a face-to-face meeting to inform these people that you no longer wish to spend time with them. Fortunately, the universe has a wonderful way of sorting things out for you. If you feel that someone is not bringing anything of value to your life and in fact the opposite, they are bringing you down, just stop spending time with them. Most people just work their way naturally out of your life when you put less energy into your relationship with them. If someone just "doesn't get it," then you may need to be more direct.

Promote: It's time to step it up a notch with these people. Tell them how much you value them and do something nice for them. Take them out for tea, write them a letter—whatever it is, show them how much they mean to you and then spend more time with them.

Clean Beauty Smoothie

This smoothie is full of detoxifying plant compounds, including chlorophyll, fiber and antioxidants. A healthy glow is the result of a detoxified body, and this smoothie will help you get your glow on!

Makes 1 smoothie

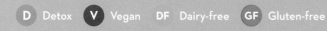 **D** Detox **V** Vegan **DF** Dairy-free **GF** Gluten-free

1 cup (250 mL) firmly packed leafy greens such as spinach, kale or collards

½ cup (125 mL) loosely packed fresh flat-leaf parsley or mint leaves

1 apple (unpeeled if organic), cored and cut in pieces

½ cup (125 mL) pineapple

Optional: ¼ cup (60 mL) hemp seeds (or 1 scoop protein powder)

In a blender, combine all ingredients with 2¼ cups (550 mL) filtered water; blend until smooth. If the smoothie is too thick, add a little more water.

5

SUPERFOODS AND HEALTHY LIFESTYLE HABITS FOR JOYOUS HEALTH

As I mentioned in the introduction of this book, more than a decade ago, when I thought I was eating healthfully, I was plagued by a hormonal imbalance that had a whole host of unpleasant effects. How did I change my life around? While working with a nutritionist, I tweaked my diet (I did not calorie count ever), chose lifestyle habits that reinforced my commitment to joyous health and, of course, added superfoods. A "new me" was born!

As I was going through this process of change, each day I felt stronger and more energized. Changes occurred that I was not expecting. My hair became shinier and my skin glowed. These results alone kept me on track. I felt amazing on the inside, and my joyous health choices were finally being reflected on the outside.

In this chapter, you will learn the superfoods, super supplements and super lifestyle habits I recommend for joyous health. Hundreds of my clients have experienced joyous health, weight loss and improvement of all their health concerns while indulging in superfoods. Healthy can and should be done deliciously!

Eat Superfoods

Now more than ever, we need to infuse our body with foods that are packed with nutrients and offer the body benefits not found in the Standard American Diet but necessary for truly joyous health.

Superfoods are not a gimmick or a trend. Many of these foods fly off store shelves once people realize the incredible potential for joyous health they offer. Some of these foods have been around for thousands of years, and for good reason. Many have medicinal benefits, high nutritional status and the ability to help you transform your health. What's more, we're not talking exotic for all foods. Many of these foods can be found in your local grocery store and perhaps even grow locally.

Intensive farming practices over the last eighty years have seriously depleted our soils of minerals such as potassium, magnesium, calcium, selenium and chromium. These nutrients not only help to prevent cancer but also aid blood sugar metabolism, which in turn helps to prevent type 2 diabetes and keep your heart healthy. And this barely scratches the surface of the benefits of these nutrients.

Why does nutrient depletion happen to soil? It's pretty straightforward. One of the most common causes is what's called monocropping. Big farms grow the exact same type of crop year after year after year. The result? The soil becomes nutrient-deficient. For example, if cauliflower is always grown in the same field, the plants will deplete the soil of the nutrients cauliflower needs most to grow and flourish. The health of the soil determines the health of the plant that grows in that soil. If you have soil that is weak, you have plants that are weak and susceptible to diseases and pests. What do these mega-farms do to counter the problem? They drown their soil and their produce in chemicals to help the plants grow and to fight off diseases and pests.

Growing a variety of crops and rotating them in a field is critical to the health of the soil. If you have soil that is healthy, you have plants that are healthy and full of nutrients. Because organic farms rotate crops and thereby naturally nourish their soils, I am committed to buying certified organic foods as often as possible.

I also prefer my fruits and vegetables without a side of pesticides, another reason I choose organic. The "Dirty Dozen" list on page 105 shows the fruits and vegetables with the highest levels of pesticides. These are the ones it's most important to buy organic. However, organic food may not always be available or within your budget, so alongside the "Dirty Dozen" you will see the "Clean 15." These are the fifteen fruits and vegetables that it's okay to buy non-organic because they have the lowest levels of pesticide contamination.

Since the average North American is eating plenty of refined foods such as white pasta, white rice and white bread that have been stripped of nutrients, as well as fruits and vegetables that contain far less nutrition than they did fifty years ago due to these mega-farms, I recommend eating superfoods. While I'm not suggesting you eat a superfood at every single meal and snack, I do recommend introducing a new superfood to your diet each week. I've found that most people need to transition into a new, healthy way of eating slowly; otherwise it's difficult to maintain. For example, you could simply add dried cranberries instead of goji berries to your trail mix (see my Superfood Trail Mix recipe on page 215) or slice up an organic apple, slather on some almond butter and sprinkle with cinnamon—both snacks have superfood status.

Why Superfoods?

Every time we turn on the television or read the newspaper, we are bombarded with depressing stats on ill health and disease taking over our nation. In 2012, nine Canadians died from cancer every single hour. More than 20 million Canadians suffer from digestive problems every year. Statistics like these are showing us that the way we are currently eating and living our lives is not working. We are getting sicker and sicker. The most ironic part is that in Canada and the United States, people have an abundance of food but are completely undernourished. There is no lack of food, just a lack of nutrients. The power is in *your* hands. You can choose to be another statistic or not.

Joyous Tip

Food is more than just fuel. The food you eat can move you closer and closer to disease—or closer and closer to joyous health. Think of the food you eat as more than simply "fuel." In fact, your skin completely renews itself every twenty-eight days. Therefore, food is literally the raw materials from which we create new cells.

What Defines a Superfood?

Before I share my favorite superfoods, let's take a quick look at the reasons some foods deserve superfood status.

High Level of Antioxidants

Highly reactive, unstable molecules called free radicals from pesticides, industrial chemicals and pollution, and even produced by your body as a byproduct of metabolism, can damage your cells and may even lead to cancer. Antioxidants are able to neutralize free radicals, preventing damage to your cells. These cancer-fighting plant medicines are found in abundance in fruits and vegetables.

A study in the July 2006 issue of the *American Journal of Clinical Nutrition* looked at the antioxidant content of foods commonly eaten in the United States. The following foods had a high level of antioxidants (listed highest to lowest):

- blackberries
- walnuts
- strawberries
- artichokes (cooked)
- cranberries
- raspberries
- blueberries
- ground cloves
- prunes
- red cabbage (cooked)
- pineapple
- oranges
- red plums
- pinto beans
- spinach (frozen)
- kiwifruit
- red potatoes
- sweet potatoes
- red peppers (cooked)
- broccoli (cooked)

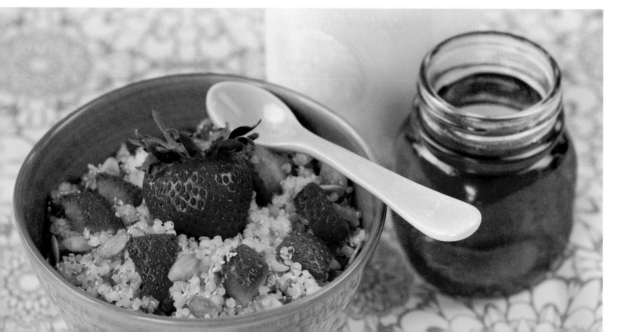

High Level of Minerals

Superfoods are a rich source of common minerals, including calcium, magnesium, phosphorus, potassium, sodium iron, selenium, iodine, copper, manganese, chromium and zinc. Of course, they contain more minerals than these, but these are the most common ones. They are essential for cardiovascular health, mental health, detoxification, prevention of disease and more. Mineral deficiencies are more common than vitamin deficiencies because our body does not manufacture any minerals and some foods are artificially enriched with vitamins.

High Level of Vitamins

Superfoods are naturally rich sources of vitamins, which are vital to the health of your cells and act mainly as coenzymes (meaning in collaboration with enzymes) in a variety of metabolic reactions in our body. But let's go a bit deeper. Vitamins have diverse essential functions in the body. Some function as antioxidants, such as vitamin E and sometimes vitamin C. Some have hormone-like functions, such as vitamin D, or are needed for tissue growth, such as some forms of vitamin A. Vitamins are essential for growth, vitality, digestion, elimination and resistance to disease. They help us stay beautiful and feel alive and vibrant.

Most vitamins cannot be made by your body, with the exception of B vitamins, which can be made by intestinal bacteria. When our diet is poor and we become deficient in any one vitamin or mineral, our bodies will provide us with signs that may be subtle, such as cracks in the corner of the mouth indicating a B_2 deficiency, or severe, such as rickets in the case of severe vitamin D deficiency or beriberi in the case of vitamin B_1 deficiency.

Keep in mind that, as nutty as it sounds, the dietary recommendations set by the government are designed merely to prevent levels of deficiency that would cause severe problems, such as rickets from vitamin D deficiency. These guidelines are not based on the amounts you need to thrive and have joyous health. I want you to thrive, not just survive or narrowly escape deficiency! Your body will provide you with symptoms of deficiency *long* before it is completely bankrupt. This is why it's important to choose foods that offer high levels of vitamins and minerals.

Beyond antioxidants, vitamins and minerals, scientists are discovering more plant medicines every day. We already know that kale contains more than forty-five flavonoids, and US Department of Agriculture researchers found that 1 cup of wild blueberries contains more than thirteen thousand antioxidants.

Top 12 Superfoods for Joyous Health

These are some of my favorite superfoods that offer a high level of nutrients and are equally delicious:

1. bee products: raw honey, royal jelly, bee pollen and propolis
2. berries (dark): blackberries, blueberries, raspberries and goji berries
3. chia seeds
4. coconut oil
5. ginger
6. hemp seeds
7. kale
8. herbs and spices: garlic, basil, rosemary, cilantro, parsley, oregano, thyme, turmeric, cinnamon, cardamom, nutmeg, cloves and ginger
9. pumpkin seeds (and squash seeds)
10. quinoa
11. raw cacao
12. spirulina

Bee Products: Raw Honey, Royal Jelly, Bee Pollen and Propolis

Years ago, I interviewed a few Ontario bee farmers. Ever since then, I've been sharing the benefits of bee products with my clients and anyone who will listen to spread my love for honey.

Honey superfoods are as ancient as they come. As far back as 5500 BCE, the Egyptians wrote about honey's benefits, and it's been used in Ayurvedic medicine in India for at least four thousand years. Clearly, I'm not the only honey lover!

But raw honey is not the only bee-produced superfood. There's also royal jelly, bee pollen and propolis.

ROYAL JELLY

Royal jelly is a milky substance secreted from the glands of worker bees and fed to all larvae in the colony and the queen bee, who lives almost exclusively off royal jelly—lucky lady. Royal jelly is the world's richest source of vitamin B_5, which is known to combat the negative effects of stress, including fatigue and insomnia, and is essential for healthy hair. Royal jelly is also anti-inflammatory and cancer preventing. In one study, mice that were injected with cancer cells showed a drastic reduction in the spread of those cells when they were also injected with royal jelly.

How to enjoy it: Royal jelly tastes very bitter, so it's best enjoyed when mixed with some raw honey and spread on a cracker. (Try the Almond Flour Rosemary Crackers on page 222.)

BEE POLLEN

Bee pollen is one of nature's best-kept secrets. Some experts believe it's one of the most complete foods because it's an excellent source of amino acids and enzymes. Pollen is a collection of little yellow granules that bees gather from flowering plants. Ironically, it has been known to be highly effective at combating allergies— fight pollen allergies with pollen!

How to enjoy it: Bee pollen can be taken in capsules, but the granules are my preference. The granules should have some variation in their yellow color. This indicates pollen from various sources, which provides a broader range of nutrients. Sprinkle it on salad, mix it into yogurt or toss it into a smoothie. Pure, raw honey is also an excellent natural source of bee pollen.

PROPOLIS

Propolis is a glue-like substance that bees collect from trees and plants to hold the hive together. Bees use it as a natural antibiotic to protect their hive and as a defense against disease. These benefits translate to human health as well: propolis has been reported to strengthen our immune system. Research shows that taking propolis during cold and flu season reduces your cold symptoms. Because of its anti-inflammatory action, it has been used to treat arthritis, allergies and asthma.

Joyous Tip

Honey: Never heat or bake with any honey product, as it can destroy the enzymes and nutrients that give honey products superfood status.

How to enjoy it: Think of propolis more as a superfood supplement than as a food you eat. You can find it in most health food stores as a tablet, capsule, powder or extract. It can be used topically as an antibiotic. It's also an ingredient in many personal care products, such as ointments and lotions. People who are allergic to bees or honey products may want to avoid these products.

Berries

Berries, especially dark ones, are nature's perfect candy! Why bother with commercial candy full of dyes, artificial flavorings and chemicals when we have an abundance of berries available to us fresh, dried and in frozen form? Berries that I recommend for joyous health include blackberries, mulberries, blueberries, goji berries, raspberries and strawberries.

JOYOUS FACTS ABOUT BERRIES

Extremely high level of flavonoids. It's flavonoids that give berries their rich color. These plant medicines are anti-inflammatory and provide both cardiovascular support and anti-aging support. A study from the *Journal of Nutrition* showed that women who consumed flavonoid-rich food saw improved skin hydration as well.

Nutrient-dense. Berries are a great source of vitamin C and B-complex vitamins. In fact, just eight strawberries has more vitamin C than one orange.

Balance blood sugar. Berries provide a slow release of glucose into the blood because their fiber slows down digestion. This high fiber content also helps prevent carb/sugar cravings.

Brain-loving. Eating berries regularly can reduce the risk of Alzheimer's disease because the protective antioxidants in berries combat the effects of stress on the brain.

Good for eye health. Studies show that eating berries improves vision and reduces age-related vision loss and cataracts.

How to enjoy them: Eat them one by one! Or try my Blueberry Spelt Pancakes (page 147) or Goji Berry Glory Muffins (page 140).

Joyous Tip

Organic on a budget? Organic berries can be expensive when they're not in season. Buy extra when they are in season and freeze them so you can enjoy them all year round. I really enjoy frozen berries in a morning smoothie—such a wonderful way to start the day!

Chia Seeds

People ask me this all the time, so yes, these are the same seeds responsible for the infamous Chia Pet from the 1980s. Chia seeds belong to the mint family and are completely gluten-free. Don't let their size (or Chia Pet past) fool you, because they are nutritional powerhouses.

JOYOUS FACTS ABOUT CHIA SEEDS

Excellent source of good fat. Chia seeds are a concentrated source of the omega-3 fatty acid alpha-linolenic acid—even higher than flaxseeds. Omega-3 fats help to lower inflammation and keep your brain and cardiovascular system healthy.

Balance blood sugar and crush cravings. One ounce of chia seeds contains 10.7 g of fiber. This highly digestible fiber slows the release of glucose into the bloodstream and gives you the sensation of fullness much faster than eating a bowl of bran cereal will. Also, keeping insulin in check will help reduce belly fat.

Complete source of protein. Chia seeds are particularly high in tryptophan, the amino acid precursor of serotonin (the happy hormone) and melatonin (the sleep/anti-cancer hormone).

Nutrient-dense. This wee powerhouse of a seed is a source of calcium, magnesium, manganese, iron, phosphorus and folic acid. These nutrients are important for cardiovascular health, bone health, stress reduction, baby making and more.

How to enjoy them: You must try the Overnight Strawberry Chia Pudding (page 157) for breakfast or for a healthy sweet treat. You can also use chia seeds as a substitute for eggs in a recipe; sprinkle them on yogurt, in cereal or in your smoothie; or use them to thicken sauces. The uses of chia are endless. I use them in many of the recipes in this book and on my Joyous Health blog.

Joyous Tip

Chia versus flax: You don't have to grind chia seeds the way you do flaxseeds. Your stomach acids break down chia seeds very easily. (If you don't grind flaxseeds to release the healthy fats, they pass right through you and down la toilette.) Sprouted chia is even better than the whole seed because it's even more digestible and higher in some vitamins, such as the B-complex.

Coconut Oil

Years ago coconut oil was unfairly demonized because of its high level of saturated fat. Harvard researchers later reviewed that initial study and concluded it was not accurate because the oil used in the study that raised cholesterol levels in rats was hydrogenated, which altered it to the point of its being devoid of *any* essential fatty acids. In fact, research shows that coconut oil not only causes an increase in HDL (good) cholesterol but also does *not* increase LDL (bad) cholesterol. And this is just one of its many health benefits.

Coconut oil has been around a long time. Hindu scriptures dating back to 1500 BCE say it nourishes the body, increases strength and promotes beautiful hair and skin. In Ayurvedic medicine, it has been used for over four thousand years as an effective treatment for skin diseases.

JOYOUS FACTS ABOUT COCONUT OIL

Contains good fats. Approximately 60 percent of the fats in coconut oil are medium-chain fatty acids (MCFAs), including lauric acid, caprylic acid and capric acid. Lauric acid accounts for as much as 75 percent of the fatty acids in coconut oil. Lauric acid is the same fat that is in breast milk, which makes it immune-building and healing. This fat is digested very easily and sent to the liver to be used as energy rather than being stored as fat.

Promotes weight loss. Studies have shown that when coconut oil is part of one's diet, white fat stores are reduced. White fat in excess around the abdominal region promotes heart disease, diabetes and many other metabolic diseases. Because MCFAs are well absorbed and used as an energy source, burning MCFAs actually increases the metabolic rate. One study showed that a diet high in MCFAs increased metabolic rate (hello, fat burning!) by 50 percent over a six-day period. That's a huge amount of fat-burning potential you can add to your smoothie!

The "anti" trio: anti-bacterial, anti-viral and anti-fungal agent.

Beautifying. You can literally slather your body in coconut oil after a shower or a bath and use it as a hair moisturizer and not have to worry about any toxic chemicals being absorbed into your bloodstream through your skin. Coconut oil is wonderful for dry, flaky and dull-looking skin or a dry scalp. It can also be used for psoriasis, dermatitis, eczema and other skin infections. I use it to keep the frizzies in my hair away and to moisturize my hands and cuticles.

Joyous Tip

High smoke point: Most vegetable oils, such as sunflower and safflower, cannot be heated; otherwise they can damage your body at a cellular level. Coconut oil's high smoke point makes it ideal for sautéing and stir-frying vegetables. Don't be afraid of using coconut oil for savory dishes. It adds a really nice flavor and is not overpowering.

Ginger

Ginger is one of my favorite ingredients to add some zippy zing to my morning fresh juice or some sautéed veggies. Ginger is more than just zippy zing, mind you. It's most famous for the anti-bloat effects it has on your belly and its anti-inflammatory benefits.

JOYOUS FACTS ABOUT GINGER

Makes your belly joyous! Gingerol, one of the main phytonutrients in ginger, helps to relax the muscles of the gastrointestinal lining, thereby preventing gas and bloating.

Anti-inflammatory gem. Gingerol is also a potent antioxidant that has been found in studies to relieve osteo- and rheumatoid arthritis pain, even in patients who didn't respond to medications. In fact, studies have shown that it reduces certain hormones that promote inflammation. Gingerol does the same job as non-steroidal anti-inflammatory drugs, but without the negative side effects such as nausea, vomiting, diarrhea and constipation.

Immune booster. During flu season, stock up on ginger because it boosts your immune system by inducing sweating, which is an excellent way to detox naturally. Remember, a fever is a sign that your immune system is fighting an infection.

Natural antibiotic. Ginger kills pathogenic bacteria, which is one of the reasons you get pickled ginger with your sushi. Be careful because this ginger often contains sulfites, which are a common food sensitivity.

How to enjoy it: Add a thumb-sized amount of ginger to a fresh juice (see recipes on page 174) or slice off a chunk and infuse it in hot water with some fresh lemon and raw honey for an immune-boosting hot drink.

Hemp Seeds (aka Hemp Hearts)

Not to be confused with their cousins, the "other" hemp seeds used to grow marijuana, these completely legal and delicious soft-textured seeds taste a bit like sunflower seeds or pine nuts.

JOYOUS FACTS ABOUT HEMP SEEDS

Complete source of vegetarian protein. Hemp seeds contain all nine essential amino acids found in animal foods and twenty amino acids in total, making them a wonderful choice for people who don't eat animal foods. In fact, a 3 tbsp (45 mL) serving of hemp hearts contains 10 g of easy-to-digest protein. Compared with soybeans, hemp contains far fewer trypsin inhibitors, which may block the absorption of protein (one of the many problems with soy). Another reason to love the easily digested protein in hemp: all those amino acids in hemp are building blocks for neurotransmitters such as feel-good dopamine and serotonin.

Source of essential fatty acids. Essential fatty acids, also known as "good fats," are the ones you need to eat because your body cannot make them. Hemp is one of the best plant-based sources of omega-3 fats. In fact, hemp seeds have a higher amount of omega-3 fats than flaxseeds do.

Unique source of gamma-linolenic acid. This fatty acid helps to balance hormones and lower inflammation ("your internal fire"). This lowered inflammation keeps your ticker joyous too! A 2008 study published in the *Canadian Journal of Physiology and Pharmacology* found that the high content of gamma-linolenic acid (GLA) in hemp seeds contributed to their ability to reduce heart disease. Numerous studies have shown that GLA has far-reaching joyous health benefits, and I have seen many of these first-hand in my practice. A good intake of GLA balances hormones, which in turn reduces PMS symptoms and menopausal hot flashes and may help with arthritis symptoms, attention deficit disorder and skin conditions such as eczema.

How to enjoy them:

You can sprinkle hemp seeds over salad, mix them into cereal or yogurt, add them to baking recipes, or simply eat them straight from the bag with a spoon— my favorite way!

Packed with nutrients. If all this wasn't enough, hemp seeds are a source of antioxidants, fiber, iron, zinc, carotene, phospholipids, phytosterols, vitamins B_1, B_2, B_6, D and E, chlorophyll, calcium, magnesium, sulfur, copper, potassium, phosphorus and enzymes. That's a whole lot of nutritional benefit in those little seeds!

Other hemp products with excellent nutritional benefits include cold-pressed hemp seed oil, hemp protein powder and my Hemp Seed Maple Cinnamon Butter (see recipe on page 220). You can also try my metabolism-boosting, craving-crushing Hemp Seed Guacamole (page 210). Thanks to the protein hit from the hemp seeds, it's a satisfying mid-afternoon snack.

Kale

Kale has been enjoyed for hundreds of years. It's the reigning Queen of the Greens, and deservedly so! Kale's high levels of fiber and nutrients will help keep your appetite in check and your blood sugar balanced.

JOYOUS FACTS ABOUT KALE

Trio of beauty vitamins—A, C and K. Combined, these help the glands of the scalp produce oils that give hair that healthy, shiny glow. These oils are hair's natural moisturizers. Vitamins A and C also protect the skin's health.

Detoxifying and anti-cancer. Glucosinolates in kale play a key role in detoxification, and kale has been linked to lowering the risk of five types of cancer: bladder, breast, colon, ovary and prostate.

Anti-inflammatory. Over forty-five plant medicines called flavonoids have been identified in kale. With kaempferol and quercetin heading the list, kale's flavonoids combine both antioxidant and anti-inflammatory benefits.

Good for bone health. Kale is a wonderful source of vitamin K and calcium, both bone-building nutrients.

Contains chlorophyll. Chlorophyll is the green matter in plant foods. It is extremely detoxifying and blood-cleansing.

Aids digestion. Kale's high amount of fiber helps with regularity and lowering cholesterol.

Other notable leafy greens are Swiss chard, collard, watercress, spinach, arugula, cabbage and green leafy lettuce. Be sure to buy organic, because conventionally grown leafy greens are sprayed with lots of pesticides.

How to enjoy it: Toss a handful into a smoothie (see page 164) or try one of the kale chip recipes on pages 206 and 208.

Herbs and Spices: Garlic, Basil, Rosemary, Cilantro, Parsley, Oregano, Thyme, Turmeric, Cinnamon, Cardamom, Nutmeg, Cloves and Ginger

There is no limit to the number of health benefits from these herbs and spices. Some of the benefits are anti-inflammatory, cancer-preventative, anti-viral, heart-healthy, immune-building and metabolism-boosting.

How to enjoy them: Add one or two of these herbs or spices to at least one meal each day. These herbs and spices are used throughout the recipes in this book.

Pumpkin Seeds (and Squash Seeds)

Pumpkin seeds, also known as pepitas, are the perfect balance of sweet and bitter tasting. They are a source of protein, omega-3 fats and antioxidant minerals and vitamins.

JOYOUS FACTS ABOUT PUMPKIN SEEDS

Skin-beautifying zinc. Pumpkin seeds are best known for their zinc content, which is what makes them a beautifying food. Zinc promotes cell division, cell repair and cell growth, all of which equate to skin health. A deficiency in zinc may result in lowered taste and smell (two of life's simplest pleasures) and can lead to acne.

Megadose of anti-aging vitamin E. Pumpkin seeds are unique in that they contain a wide variety of vitamin E forms: alpha-tocopherol, gamma-tocopherol, delta-tocopherol, alpha-tocomonoenol and gamma-tocomonoenol. The last two forms are very easily absorbed by the body and are not frequently found in foods. Vitamin E is a powerful anti-aging antioxidant because it protects our cells from free-radical damage that may otherwise age our skin. However, supplementation may not achieve the same results as eating the whole food. Instead of popping pills or buying a $60 bottle of anti-aging cream, eat some pumpkin seeds!

Heart health and women's health. Pumpkin seeds are rich in magnesium, which helps lower blood pressure and reduce the risk of heart attack or stroke. Magnesium is often deficient in women who suffer from PMS.

How to enjoy them: Nutrient-dense pumpkin seeds add a nice crunch as a salad topper or in a trail mix (see recipe on page 215) to increase the protein and antioxidant content. They can also be brewed as a tea decoction to treat intestinal worms (especially roundworm and tapeworm): simply add 3 tbsp (45 mL) of seeds to 1 cup (250 mL) of boiling water, simmer for 15 minutes, then strain. Buy pumpkin seeds raw and unsalted and be sure to refrigerate them. Give them a sniff before you eat them—they should not smell rancid. Sunflower and sesame seeds are also joyous.

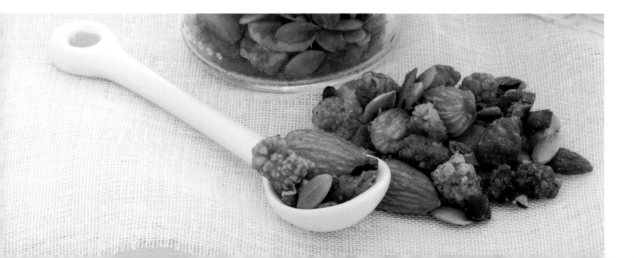

Quinoa

The United Nations declared 2013 the International Year of Quinoa. This popular ancient seed has been around since 3000 BCE and was once known as the "gold of the Aztecs" because of the strength and stamina its nutrients provide. Quinoa is cooked just like rice. It has a mild, slightly nutty flavor and is very versatile. It basically takes on the flavor of what you serve or cook it with.

JOYOUS FACTS ABOUT QUINOA

Complete protein. Just like hemp seeds, quinoa contains all the essential amino acids, which makes it a "complete" protein. It also has significantly greater amounts than other grains of both lysine (excellent at treating and preventing cold sores and promoting tissue repair) and isoleucine.

Hypoallergenic food. Quinoa is naturally gluten-free and very easy to digest, provided it's cooked properly to remove all the bitter saponins.

Nutrient-dense. Quinoa is a good source of many minerals and vitamins, including heart-healthy magnesium, manganese, iron, copper, zinc, bone-building phosphorus and the B-complex vitamins. Quinoa is unique in that it contains many members of the vitamin E tocopherol family, which are largely absent from most other grains.

Antioxidants and anti-inflammatory. Quinoa is rich in antioxidants and anti-inflammatory phytonutrients, such as ferulic acid, coumaric acid, hydroxybenzoic acid and vanillic acid. Future research will likely show us that it is a cancer-preventing food because of these nutrients.

How to enjoy it: Quinoa can be the main event of your meal or a side dish, and it works in both sweet and savory dishes. Look for quinoa flour for baking. There are many quinoa recipes in this book—check out the Curry Lentil Loaf on page 234 and learn how to make the perfect quinoa for any dish on page 137.

Quinoa can have a bitter taste because of its naturally present saponins—nature's way of protecting the seed from predators. Most store-bought quinoa has been commercially processed to remove the saponins found in the outer coat of the seed. However, you should still rinse quinoa seeds before cooking them. Place the seeds in a fine-mesh sieve and run water over them while gently rubbing them together in your hands. Taste a few seeds to determine if a bitter taste remains. Repeat this process until the quinoa no longer tastes bitter.

Joyous Tip

Seed or grain: Quinoa is often referred to as a grain or a pseudo-cereal but it's actually neither. It's a seed, and belongs to the same family as spinach, Swiss chard and beets. Quinoa is a wonderful gluten-free alternative to wheat, barley and rye.

Raw Cacao

Cacao, another ancient superfood, was once so valued by the Maya and the Aztecs that it was used as currency. You've probably heard about the health benefits of chocolate, but there's more to the story, because not all chocolate is created equal. For instance, cocoa and cacao are very different. Cocoa, although it comes from the same source as cacao, is processed with heat and offers few to no health benefits, while raw cacao is truly a superfood. Because of the stimulating nature of the caffeine and theobromine in raw cacao, be cautious when introducing this superfood to your diet if it's new to you.

How to enjoy it: My two favorite ways to enjoy cacao are by sprinkling the nibs on top of a smoothie for some crunch, and in a raw chocolate pudding (see my recipe on page 270) for an antioxidant punch. Cacao powder can be used in a smoothie (try my Raspberry Chocolate Cheesecake Smoothie on page 162), or you can get creative and make your own chocolate almond milk sweetened with stevia or coconut sugar by adding 2–3 tbsp raw cacao powder to the recipe on page 170.

JOYOUS FACTS ABOUT RAW CACAO

Chock-full of antioxidants. Cacao powder is one of the richest sources of antioxidants found in nature. There are more antioxidant flavonoids in cacao than in red wine or green tea.

Nutrient-dense. Raw cacao is rich in magnesium, and many researchers speculate that this is why women crave chocolate during PMS. Raw cacao also contains other essential minerals, among them calcium, zinc, iron, copper, sulfur and potassium.

Mood- and energy-boosting naturally occurring chemicals. All raw cacao products contain the unique alkaloid chemicals theobromine, phenylethylamine and anandamine.

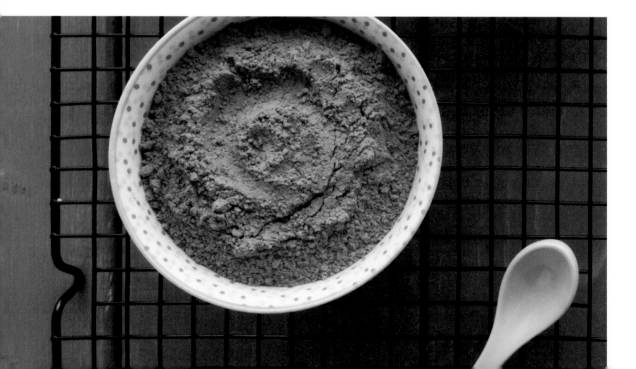

Spirulina

Spirulina is a blue-green algae that is rich in protein, vitamins, minerals and antioxidants. Spirulina is often considered one of the most nutritious foods available.

Complete protein. By weight, spirulina contains 60 to 70 percent protein. Just like hemp and quinoa, it is a source of complete protein.

Balances blood sugar. Because of its high level of protein, spirulina can help to stabilize blood sugar when it is used as a supplement between meals and can help to reduce sugar fluctuations in type 2 diabetes and in those with hypoglycemia.

Contains energizing B vitamins. Spirulina is a good source of vitamins B_1, B_2, B_3, B_6 and B_9 (folic acid). Many companies claim that spirulina is a source of vitamin B_{12}, but this type of B_{12} in spirulina is inactive in the human body, so other sources or supplementation is still required.

Blood-building and detoxifying. Chlorophyll is what gives spirulina its gorgeous green color. Interestingly, chlorophyll strongly resembles the human hemoglobin molecule—the one that carries oxygen in the bloodstream—so it's not surprising that chlorophyll is nourishing for the red blood cells. It's also a potent detoxifier: it speeds the release of toxins from the bloodstream by binding with those toxins in the intestines.

How to enjoy it: Spirulina is not a food that you eat on its own because it's not very tasty. One of my favorite greens superfood powders, Greens+ O by Genuine Health, contains 1450 mg of spirulina per scoop, with a variety of other nutrients and stevia to sweeten it. The best way to eat spirulina is by adding it to yogurt or a smoothie. You can simply mix it with water if you wish. I even know some raw vegan chefs who make cheesecake (no cheese, obviously) with it.

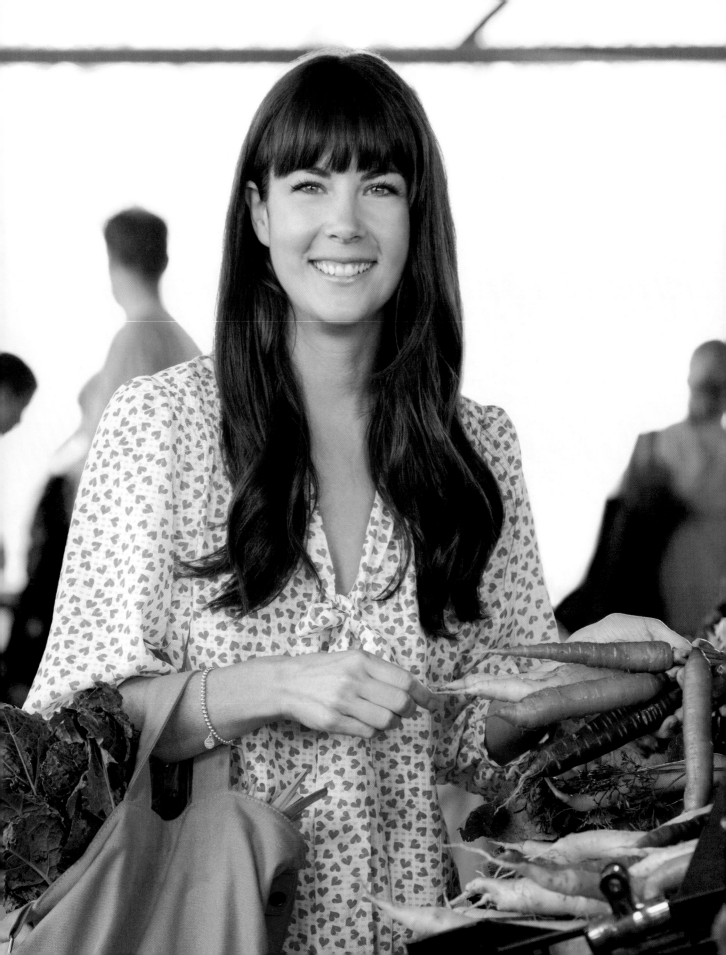

Eat a Rainbow of Colors

When it comes to the food we eat, color is a cue for joyous health. That's because many of the pigments that fruits and vegetables get their vibrant color from are considered phytonutrients—natural chemicals found in plants. Different colors offer up different phytonutrients with a variety of health benefits.

Science proves this. A study from Colorado State University found that subjects who ate several different phytonutrients from a wide variety of fruits and vegetables experienced lower levels of DNA oxidation (an indication of free-radical damage) compared with those who ate larger amounts of only a handful of plant foods and, therefore, a more limited spectrum of antioxidants. Fill your grocery cart with a rainbow of cheery colors, because the more diverse, the better.

One of my first clients, Amanda, told me she had the healthiest diet and yet was plagued with health issues, specifically low energy and digestive problems. When I reviewed her food journal, I found that she had been eating the exact same foods for several years. Every day she ate blueberries on top of a processed cereal for breakfast, trail mix for a snack, tuna on a whole wheat wrap for lunch, and for dinner she always had a smoothie with some of the superfoods listed above, but she was eating the same foods every day. Her diet lacked variety, and this was why she had health problems in addition to food sensitivities caused by eating the same foods day after day. Once she got some more colors and variety into her diet, her symptoms vanished. So vary what you eat!

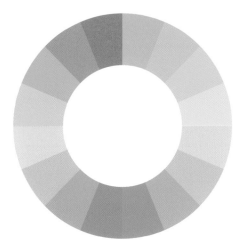

RED Red-hued foods such as pink and red grapefruit, tomatoes (especially tomato paste) and watermelon contain lycopene, the powerful pigment and carotenoid that has gained attention for its cancer-fighting ability.

ORANGE/YELLOW Orange- and yellow-fleshed vegetables and fruits such as sweet potatoes, carrots, winter squash and apricots are full of the carotenoid antioxidant beta-carotene. Many studies show that these color pigments reduce the risk of cardiovascular disease because of their ability to protect cells from damage caused by free radicals. These orange pigments also enhance the immune system and protect your skin.

GREEN Green vegetables such as spinach, kale and Swiss chard provide a healthy dose of lutein and zeaxanthin, a dynamic antioxidant duo shown to bolster eye and heart health.

BLUE Blue-colored fruits and vegetables such as blueberries, grapes, black currants, blackberries and red cabbage are a source of anthocyanins. These dark-tinted foods may protect the brain from free radicals and improve brain function, including memory.

Keep in mind that you are not limited to just the superfoods I've highlighted here. There are plenty more out there! In fact, I could probably write an entire book just on the benefits of various superfoods. Other notable superfoods include:

- apples
- avocados
- acai powder
- beans and lentils
- broccoli
- Brussels sprouts
- camu camu powder
- cauliflower
- cranberries (dried)
- extra-virgin olive oil
- fatty fish: salmon and sardines
- fermented foods: sauerkraut, kefir and kombucha
- flaxseeds
- grapes
- green tea
- maca root
- plant-based protein powders such as Genuine Health Vegan Proteins+ and Sunwarrior brand
- rooibos tea
- root vegetables such as carrots, beets and parsnips
- sacha inchi seeds
- walnuts
- white tea

Avoiding Pesticides in Fruits and Vegetables

The following list was revised by the Environmental Working Group in 2013 based on forty-three thousand tests to assess the level of pesticides found on fruits and vegetables. The "Dirty Dozen" lists the fruits and vegetables found to have the highest levels of pesticide residue. The list was expanded with a "Plus" category in 2012 to include two crops—summer squash and leafy greens (kale and collard greens). I like to refer to it as the "Filthy 14."

Dirty Dozen Plus

These foods are listed from highest level of pesticides to lowest. Keep in mind that despite sweet bell peppers being number 12, that's still high compared with the produce on the "Clean 15."

1. apples
2. celery
3. cherry tomatoes
4. cucumbers
5. grapes
6. hot peppers
7. nectarines (imported)

8. peaches
9. potatoes
10. spinach
11. strawberries
12. sweet bell peppers

Plus: kale and collard greens; summer squash (zucchini)

Source: Environmental Working Group, www.ewg.org/foodnews.

In government tests analyzed by the Environmental Working Group, 68 percent of food samples had detectable pesticide residues even *after* they had been washed or peeled. While washing will remove some pesticides, clearly it's not enough. Plus the peel contains most of the nutrients, so peeling an apple, for example, is a waste of money and valuable nutrition. You can substantially lower your pesticide exposure by purchasing organic versions of the Dirty Dozen foods.

The good news! Here is the Environmental Working Group's list of the fruits and vegetables, called the "Clean 15," found to have the lowest levels of pesticides. These are safe to eat non-organic.

Clean 15

1. asparagus
2. avocados
3. cabbage
4. cantaloupe
5. sweet corn
6. eggplant
7. grapefruit
8. kiwifruit

9. mangoes
10. mushrooms
11. onions
12. papayas
13. pineapples
14. sweet peas (frozen)
15. sweet potatoes

Source: Environmental Working Group, www.ewg.org/foodnews.

5 Super-Joyous Lifestyle Habits

This book would not be complete if I did not include a section on lifestyle habits for joyous health. From a holistic perspective, it's not just about what you eat; it's also about how you live your life, the thoughts you think and how often you move your beautiful body and engage in activities that promote balance and keep stress levels in check. These are my top recommendations to help you achieve and maintain joyous health.

1. Get a Daily Dose of Vitamin G

My parents live in a very rural area—or as I usually call it, the sticks. Whenever I spend time at their home surrounded by nature, I feel incredibly relaxed and rejuvenated. This is thanks to vitamin G, otherwise known as greenspace. Get the nature vitamin, vitamin G, as often as you possibly can.

The term "vitamin G" was used by the authors of *Your Brain on Nature*, Dr. Eva Selhub and naturopath Dr. Alan Logan, in relation to something they called ecotherapy—a belief that patient care should include time spent outdoors. I know you probably don't need a study to convince you that greenspace makes you feel joyous, but for the science-minded, here's just one example (of the proof) from the book.

Researcher Robert Ulrich evaluated eleven years' worth of data from a single suburban Pennsylvania hospital. He collected data involving adults who had undergone identical surgery to remove the gallbladder. The major distinction among the patients was the room they recovered in. One wing had windows with a view of a mini forest, while the other wing had a view of red bricks. Those patients viewing the mini forest required less potent pain medications and were found to have significantly shorter hospital stays, fewer post-surgical complaints and fewer negative comments written in their charts by nurses.

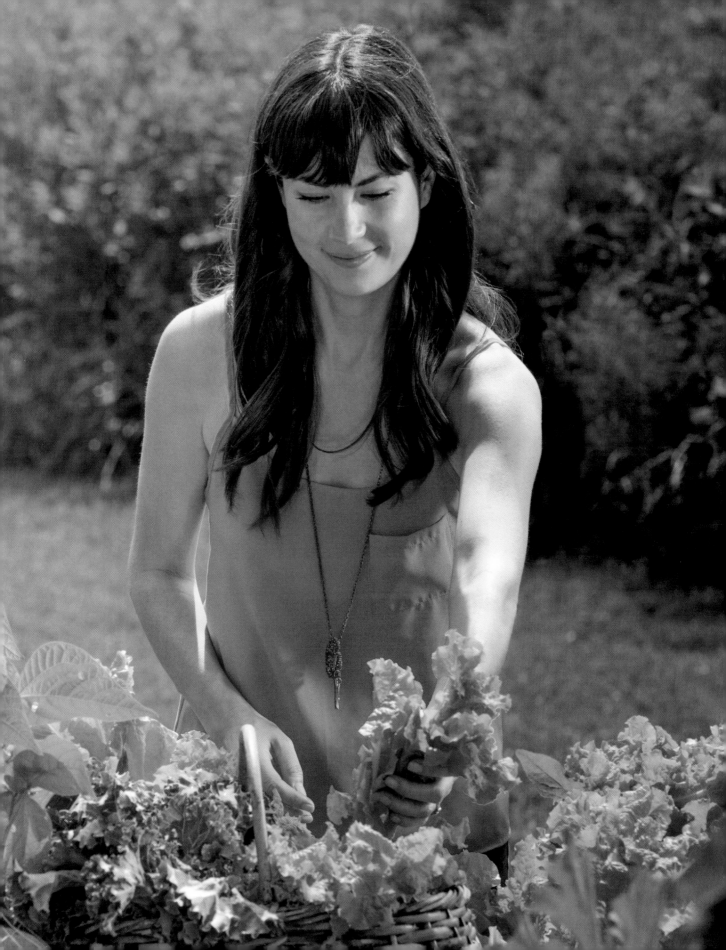

No, this doesn't mean hiking through a forest naked, but I won't hold you back from doing that as well! As explained in *Your Brain on Nature*, *shinrin-yoku* is the concept of "forest bathing," which was introduced in 1982 by the Forest Agency of Japan. *Shinrin-yoku* studies involved over a thousand subjects in twenty-four different forest settings. The research found that spending time and exercising in a forest setting can decrease psychological stress, depressive symptoms and hostility, as well as increase vigor and a feeling of liveliness. Forest bathing was also found to result in a reduction in cortisol, blood pressure and pulse rate, and an increase in immune system function.

One of the reasons this happens is that trees release chemicals called phytoncides, which can lower the production of stress hormones, reduce anxiety and increase pain tolerance.

It may not always be possible to be in nature every day if you live in a big city, but do make an effort at least once a week to forest bathe and get your dose of vitamin G!

2. Get the Music Mineral

I love music. It helps me to exercise more intensely, relaxes me when I'm stuck in traffic and has the power to lift my spirit and inspire me. Apparently, I'm not the only one deeply affected by music. According to researchers at McGill University, the brain is a very musical organ.

Just as minerals are essential to brain health, scientists have found that listening to music releases dopamine, a neurotransmitter in the brain linked to tangible, reward-related pleasures such as food, drugs and sex. Music, therefore, is like a mineral! A study from the Montreal Neurological Institute and Hospital reveals that even the anticipation of pleasurable music induces dopamine release. Translation: music makes you feel joyous!

Music is good for kids, too. A study published in the *Journal of Neuroscience* in 2013 suggests that musical training before the age of seven has a significant effect on the development of the brain. Study participants who began training early had stronger connections between motor regions—the parts of the brain that help you plan and carry out movements.

You can listen to music anywhere. I highly recommend a daily dose of the music mineral.

3. Hug—It Releases the Love Hormone

Hugging: yet another lifestyle habit that I probably don't need to persuade you to do as often as possible, but perhaps this little fact will make you hug someone for *longer*: the average hug lasts a measly three seconds!

Twenty-second hugs, on the other hand, release oxytocin, also known as the love and bonding hormone, according to researcher Dr. Helen Fisher. This is the same hormone a mother releases after giving birth that helps her bond with her baby and facilitates milk production. Have you ever wondered why some elderly couples seem more bonded? Oxytocin is also what binds lovers together long after that initial lustful honeymoon phase of a relationship has faded. Oxytocin has many other health benefits.

- It creates feelings of calmness as it counteracts the stress hormone cortisol.
- It establishes a sense of connection and bonding.
- It reduces stress.
- It increases immunity and helps tissues repair, heal and restore faster.
- It lowers blood pressure.
- It protects against heart disease.
- It reduces cravings and addictions.
- It eases depression.

So remember, next time you hug someone, make it last at least twenty seconds!

4. Make Sleep a Priority

As mentioned in chapter 3, sleep-deprived people eat more carbs, sugars and unhealthy foods. The sleep-deprived people I see in my practice commonly complain of low energy, depression, anxiety and an inability to lose weight. This is not surprising when you consider how important this health habit is.

Lack of sleep even affects your immune system. A study published in the *Archives of Internal Medicine* in September 2006 found that chronic sleeplessness is linked to an increase in cytokine molecules that control immune response. Certain cytokines increase inflammation. When inflammation is elevated, you are at a greater risk of developing an infection.

If you want to keep your appetite in check, make sure you get adequate shut-eye. A 2004 study at the University of Chicago discovered that sleep loss could reduce the body's ability to regulate hormones that control hunger.

Lastly, you are less likely to cook your own meals when you're sleep-deprived. A study presented at a 2007 conference sponsored by the American Academy of Sleep Medicine suggested that people who don't get enough sleep are more likely to rely on restaurants and fast-food outlets for some of their meals. Eating fast food can result in nutritional deficiencies, weight gain and other health problems.

The key is to make sleep a priority. The old saying "Sleep when you're dead" is a bit misleading, since a lack of sleep can cause you to age faster. Don't neglect this incredible habit! It's free and it's beautifying, so be sure to get yourself an eye mask and hit the sack for at least seven and a half hours of sleep each night in complete darkness.

5. Practice Gratefulness

A few years ago, I had a client named Emma who hired me as her nutritionist all the way from Australia—we did her sessions on Skype. As you will see on the testimonials page of my Joyous Health blog, one of the changes Emma focused on every day was a gratefulness journal. She had incredible results and an overall improvement in her health and well-being.

Science is just catching up to the concept of gratitude, but religions and ancient philosophers have long embraced gratitude as an integral component of health and well-being, and you can benefit from it, too!

Author and researcher Dr. Robert Emmons, of the University of California, discovered the power of gratitude during eight years of intensive research on the topic, which he wrote about in his book *Thanks! How the New Science of Gratitude Can Make You Happier*. Emmons found that people who view life as a gift and consciously acquire an "attitude of gratitude" experience multiple advantages, including improved emotional and physical health and strengthened relationships. "Without gratitude, life can be lonely, depressing and impoverished," says Emmons. "Gratitude enriches human life. It elevates, energizes, inspires and transforms. People are moved, opened and humbled through expressions of gratitude."

Gratefulness is a powerful healer. I suggest that every night before bed, you write down three things you are grateful for. When you are feeling sad or lonely, or you've had a bad day, read your gratefulness journal as a reminder of all the reasons to be grateful. Sharing your gratefulness is a very joyous thing to do as well. Be sure to let others know when you are grateful for them.

Carrot Cake Smoothie

One of my absolute favorite treats growing up was carrot cake (still is!). This smoothie, with shredded carrots and spices, tastes like carrot cake—but is far better for you!

Makes 1 smoothie (about 2½ cups/625 mL)

V Vegan **DF** Dairy-free **GF** Gluten-free **J** Joyous Comfort

2 Medjool dates, pitted

¼ cup (60 mL) shredded carrots

¼ cup (60 mL) hemp seeds

1 scoop vanilla protein powder

1 to 2 tbsp (15 to 30 mL) raw honey

1 tsp (5 mL) organic pure vanilla extract

1 tsp (5 mL) cinnamon

½ tsp (2 mL) nutmeg

¼ tsp (1 mL) ground cloves

1 cup (250 mL) ice water

Coconut milk, just enough to cover dry ingredients

Place all ingredients in a high-powered blender and blend until fully combined, 30 to 60 seconds.

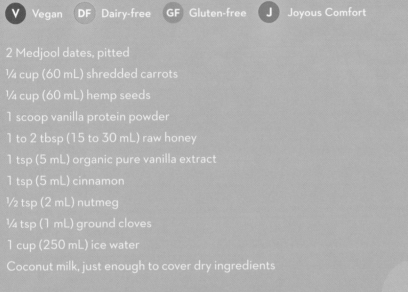

6

CREATE A JOYOUS KITCHEN

Congratulations! You've made it through the first half of *Joyous Health*, and I hope you have gained plenty of delicious knowledge. As the simple but true saying goes, If you have good food in your fridge, you will eat good food. Remember that creating a joyous kitchen doesn't have to be done in one day. Let the information in this chapter inspire you and be a springboard from which you try out new things each week.

Baby steps are key to long-term sustainable change. Transition slowly over time. Meaning, if you are currently eating mostly processed foods and very few raw foods, don't go full-force and start juicing every day. Such an all-or-nothing approach may set you up for failure. Juicing can also awaken a lot of toxic matter in the body, another reason it's best to start off just gradually incorporating more raw foods into your diet if you currently eat mostly cooked and processed foods.

When you focus on small changes over time, it's easier to keep the momentum going and easier to incorporate a new change each week. It is a far more sustainable approach. I want you to be successful, so introduce changes at your own pace. And remember that every bite is one step closer to joyous health.

All right, now it's time to create a joyous kitchen! You want to build your kitchen and stock your fridge and pantry around the Joyous Health Food Pyramid. This is truly the healthiest way of eating

Joyous Health Food Pyramid

At the top of the pyramid are foods that should be consumed in the smallest quantities, and at the bottom are foods that should be consumed in the largest quantities.

1
SWEET TREATS AND INDULGENCES

Occasionally

dark chocolate, red wine, homemade baked goods

2
PROTEIN
3 to 4 servings per day

Meat, Eggs
0 to 2 servings per day
Eggs, chicken, turkey; limit red meat or game to once per week.

Fish
1 to 2 servings per week
Check Sea Choice (www.seachoice.org) for the most sustainable options.

Nuts and Seeds
1 to 3 servings per day
Especially hemp and chia seeds— both are complete proteins.

Beans and Legumes
2 to 3 servings per day
Choose fermented soy (e.g., tempeh or miso) over tofu.

Protein Powder 1 serving per day

3
WHOLE GRAINS

2 to 3 servings per day

brown rice, wild rice, spelt, kamut, millet, quinoa, amaranth, sprouted grains

4
FRUITS

3 to 5 servings per day
dark berries, apples, pears, citrus

5
GOOD FATS AND OILS

3 to 5 servings per day

avocado, extra-virgin olive oil, flaxseed or hemp oil
Can include goat cheese if no sensitivities are present.

6
VEGETABLES

8 to 10 servings per day

kale, carrots, cauliflower, red pepper

7
WATER AND HERBAL CAFFEINE-FREE TEAS

6 to 12 glasses of water per day
(2 to 3 of these can be herbal tea)

water with lemon, cup of green tea

These foods are merely examples; do not feel limited to these items.
See pages 118–123 for a comprehensive list.

Joyous Tip

Drink up! For a more precise measurement of how much water you need to drink, divide your body weight (in pounds) in half. You should drink that number of ounces each day—or, if you're metric, multiply that number by 30 mL. For example, if you weigh 200 pounds, you should drink 100 ounces of water (or 12½ cups, which is just over eight 12-ounce glasses; or 3000 mL or 3 L). If you weigh closer to 100 pounds, you will need only about 50 ounces of water (or 1500 mL), or about four 12-ounce glasses daily. Your body will tell you what it needs if you listen. Check the color of your urine; in most cases if it's dark yellow you're likely dehydrated, and if it's pale yellow you're well hydrated.

Using the Pyramid

Don't feel constrained by the Joyous Health Food Pyramid—instead, let it guide and inspire you. There are nearly seven billion people on planet Earth and just as many different ways to eat. What makes one person feel incredible may not be the best for you. I encourage you to fine-tune any plan to suit your unique needs.

If you are new to the Joyous Health way of eating, I recommend you introduce healthier, fiber-rich foods slowly. Otherwise, a sudden increase of raw veggies may make you feel bloated and gassy. Your gut takes time to tone and adjust. It's just like starting a new exercise regimen: you don't start off doing fifty push-ups on your first day; you start with five or ten and gradually build from there.

If you suffer from any inflammatory bowel disease, you will need to modify the Joyous Health plan because raw foods and high-fiber foods may aggravate your condition. Consult with your natural healthcare practitioner before making significant changes to your diet.

· · ·

Be kind to yourself. Transition slowly.
Allow your body time to adjust to
the joyous way of eating!

· · ·

Joyous Health 10-Day Meal Plan

The recipes on this meal plan and the order in which they appear are merely suggestions. For example, you may substitute Day 2 lunch with Day 6 dinner. Interchange joyous recipes in the second half of my book as you wish!

MEAL	DAY 1	DAY 2	DAY 3	DAY 4	DAY 5	
BEFORE BREAKFAST	Fresh lemon in water or Greens+ O in water	Fresh lemon in water or Greens+ O in water	Fresh lemon in water or Greens+ O in water	Fresh lemon in water or Greens+ O in water	Fresh lemon in water or Greens+ O in water	
BREAKFAST	1 Goji Berry Glory Muffin + Morning Energizer Blueberry Smoothie	Quinoa Berry Bowl	Green Beauty Juice + Overnight Strawberry Chia Pudding	Avocado Kale Tartine + Overnight Strawberry Chia Pudding	Apple Walnut Sprouted French Toast	
LUNCH	Chickpea Detox Salad + sliced apple with Hemp Seed Maple Cinnamon Butter	Apple Beet Carrot Slaw + 5 small brown rice crackers with Hemp Seed Guacamole	Chilled Kale Walnut Pesto on brown rice pasta mixed with raw arugula or kale. Top with any dressing.	Leftover Turkey Burger + 2 cups (500 mL) leafy greens and any dressing	Apple Beet Carrot Slaw + Cardamom Parsnip Pear Soup	
DINNER	Curry Chicken Burger with Mango Salsa + mixed green salad with Keep It Simple Detox Dressing	Gluten-free pasta with Kale Walnut Pesto	1 Turkey Burger with Guac Salsa + Walker's Spicy Brussels Sprouts	Cardamom Parsnip Pear Soup + baked chicken + mixed green salad	Baked Lemon Pepper Salmon with "Cream" Sauce + ¾ cup (175 mL) Mashed Cauliflower with Goat Cheese	
SNACKS	Superfood Trail Mix	Sunshine Juice	Turmeric Sea Salt Popcorn	Cut-up veggies + tahini dip	Chocolate Protein Square	

Note: This meal plan could work over a 1- to 2-month period because leftovers can be used over a couple of days.

MEAL	DAY 6	DAY 7	DAY 8	DAY 9	DAY 10
BEFORE BREAKFAST	Fresh lemon in water or Greens+ O in water	Fresh lemon in water or Greens+ O in water	Fresh lemon in water or Greens+ O in water	Fresh lemon in water or Greens+ O in water	Fresh lemon in water or Greens+ O in water
BREAKFAST	1 Apricot Oat Granola Muffin + Green Goddess Smoothie	Sunshine Juice + Maple Banana Grilled Sandwich	1 piece of toast with Hemp Seed Maple Cinnamon Butter + Green Goddess Smoothie	1 Almond Power Muffin + fruit salad + Detox Juice	Blueberry Spelt Pancakes with Coconut Butter
LUNCH	Leftover salmon + 2 cups (500 mL) mixed green salad with any dressing	Kale Orange Pecan Salad + Hemp Seed Guacamole + organic blue corn chips	2 Raw Sunshine Wraps	Curry Lentil Loaf + Kale Chips	Summer Lovin' Gazpacho + Kale Chips + Chocolate Protein Square
DINNER	Mango Cashew Millet Salad	Amy's Tempeh Chili	Mama Bea's Curry Lentil Soup + Almond Flour Rosemary Crackers with Beet Goat Cheese Dip	Chilled Cucumber Avocado Soup + baked or grilled fish with lemon	Sun-Dried Tomato Arugula Spelt Crust Pizza + mixed green salad with Dijon Honey Dressing
SNACKS	Kale Chips	Sliced apple + Hemp Seed Butter	Fruit Salad with Cashew Orange Cream	Chewy Almond Butter Cookie + fruit	Cut-up veggies + Sun-Dried Tomato Hummus

Serving sizes: These are entirely dependent on your age, sex, level of activity and metabolism. I suggest you listen to your body and follow these tips for guidance.

- Eat when you are actually hungry—when you get that warm sensation in your belly—rather than to fill time or satisfy an emotional hunger. Listen to the cues your body gives you.

- Eat mindfully. Avoid watching TV, using your computer or talking on the phone while eating. For more mindful eating tips, see page 6.

- Eat slowly. Chew your food until it's a paste. For example, if you are eating an apple, chew until you cannot tell the difference between the flesh and the skin.

- Eat until you are 80 percent full. You'll have a good sense of this if you eat when you are actually hungry, as per the first point.

Stock Your Kitchen Joyously!

These are the foods you'll want to keep on hand in your kitchen. All these items can be found in your grocery store or health food store.

Breads/cereals/pasta: quinoa (black, red and/or white), brown rice, millet, amaranth, buckwheat, teff, steel-cut oats.

Many bread options contain a variety of gluten-free "grains." As for pasta, quinoa pasta is my preferred gluten-free pasta for flavor, but many gluten-free options are available. Make sure you avoid white rice products: even though they are gluten-free, they're still a junk food and highly processed. If you don't have any trouble digesting gluten, be sure to buy organic, stone-ground flours for baking such as spelt and kamut; people tend to react to them much less than they do wheat.

Fats and oils: Butter, clarified butter (also known as ghee), extra-virgin olive oil, coconut oil (make sure it smells like coconut), sesame oil, hemp oil, flaxseed oil and grapeseed oil are some of my favorite oils to use. Nearly all nuts and seeds can be turned into oil, so don't be surprised if you see macadamia nut or almond oil at the health food store. Just make sure it's as minimally processed as possible.

Always choose organic when you buy fats and oils. Toxins are fat-soluble, so non-organic butter is just a big glob of toxic fat! Be sure the oils you buy are cold-pressed and in a can or dark glass bottle to ensure freshness (light and exposure to air can be detrimental to oils). Avoid liquid oils in plastic bottles because chemicals in the plastic can leach into the oil.

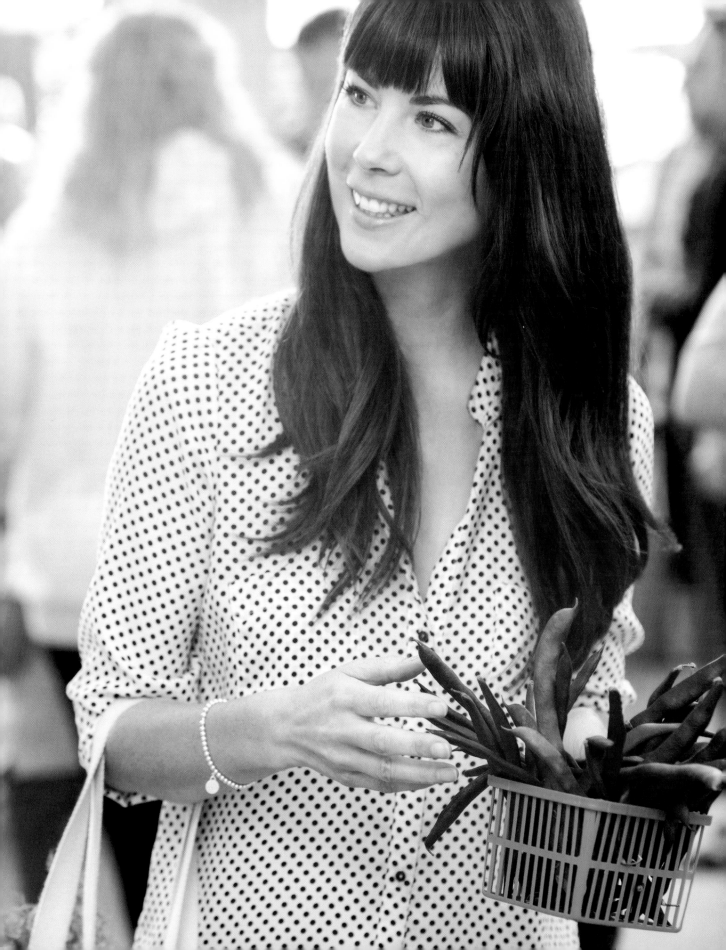

HEATING OILS

Ever wonder why some oils can be heated and others cannot? It all depends on the type of fats in a particular oil. The more saturated fat an oil contains, the more stable it is when exposed to any form of energy, such as heat, light or oxygen. As you will see below, coconut oil is nearly 90 percent saturated fat, which makes it—along with ghee and grapeseed oil—very stable at high heat. Flaxseed and olive oil are primarily monounsaturated and polyunsaturated, meaning they are less stable and more prone to break down when heated. Extra-virgin olive oil should not be heated higher than low heat, despite what you may have heard. High heat destroys all the beneficial properties of the oil, including antioxidants, and turns it rancid. The same is true for many vegetable oils, including safflower and sunflower oil. Never heat hemp or flaxseed oil. Sesame oil can be heated on a low temperature, but because its taste is very strong, I don't usually cook with it.

TYPE OF OIL	MONOUNSATURATED (%)	POLYUNSATURATED (%)	SATURATED (%)
Coconut	5.8	1.8	86.5
Flaxseed	22	74	4
Olive	77	8.4	13.5

Source: www.virgintogo.co.uk

Condiments: sea salt or Himalayan rock salt, pepper, organic balsamic vinegar, apple cider vinegar, organic Dijon mustard, raw honey, molasses, pure vanilla extract, hot sauce (no preservatives), nutritional yeast (great as a substitute for Parmesan cheese)

Spices/herbs: fresh ginger, garlic, oregano, basil, thyme, rosemary, turmeric (or curry powder), cayenne, cinnamon, cloves, allspice, nutmeg (my personal favorites, but the list is endless)

Choose fresh herbs as often as possible. Note that packaged dried spices may contain gluten.

Tea: green, white, rooibos, chamomile, peppermint

The sky is the limit! Some teas enhance detoxification, so start slowly with these ones: dandelion, burdock root, milk thistle and ginger. Many brands contain a combination of herbs, meaning tea with two or more detoxifying herbs.

Nuts and seeds: walnuts, pecans, almonds, brazil nuts, macadamia nuts, cashews, chia seeds, flaxseeds, pumpkin seeds, sesame seeds, sunflower seeds

Buy only whole, raw and unroasted nuts with no added salt. Nut and seed butters are also available. Keep all your nuts and seeds (and butters) in the fridge or freezer, as they grow mold very quickly and the fats turn rancid at a faster rate when stored at room temperature. Peanuts are heavily sprayed and can have high levels of mold, even when organic. They also tend to be a common food sensitivity and allergen. Even if you have no problems with peanut butter, you should still eat peanut products in moderation.

Joyous Tip

Increase the digestibility of your nuts. Soak your nuts in water for 3 to 4 hours or overnight before eating. This makes them more digestible because it removes the enzyme inhibitors.

Dried fruit: figs, dates, prunes, cranberries, raisins, apricots, apples

Always eat dried fruit in moderation and make sure it's labeled "sulfite-free" (see page 73). Buy dried fruit in bulk to keep costs down and always combine it with a nut or seed to lower its glycemic index (and keep your blood sugar in check).

Fruits and vegetables

Keep your fridge stocked full of fresh produce each week. Keep frozen berries on hand so you can always make a smoothie, and keep frozen vegetables for a last-minute dinner option. Choose fresh fruits and vegetables that are in season as often as possible and go for brightly colored fruits and vegetables (refer to the color chart on page 103). And remember to mix it up! Don't buy the same produce week after week.

Seaweeds: arame, dulse, hijiki, kombu, nori, wakame

I love using a nori sheet as a wrap and stuffing it with quinoa, spices and vegetables.

Animal protein: whole organic eggs, fish, chicken, quail, Cornish hen, turkey, grass-fed meat (e.g., beef, bison, lamb, wild game)

Joyous Tip

Can't eat eggs? Here's my favorite egg replacement for baking:
2 tbsp (30 mL) sprouted flax and chia + ⅓ cup (75 mL) water = 1 egg.
Let the mixture sit for a few minutes to become gelatinous.

Vegetarian protein: organic tempeh (fermented tofu), hemp seeds, chia seeds, sprouts (any sprouted bean, e.g., mung), quinoa, nuts and seeds (preferably soaked before eating), plant-based protein powders, beans and legumes (chickpeas, lentils, mung beans, white beans, black beans and navy beans are the easiest to digest). Don't forget about green vegetables! In fact, watercress is 84 percent protein and spirulina is 60 percent protein.

Cheese

Exercise caution with cheese. The protein called casein in cheese is a common food sensitivity, and a little goes a long way. Be sure to buy organic and raw when available. Goat cheese tends to be more digestible than hard cheeses such as cheddar and Swiss. When missing a good fat in their diet, many people will naturally crave cheese. Avocado is a wonderful replacement for your cheese habit, and a few slices of this buttery fruit are a nice way to change up your sandwich.

Canned foods

Keep canned food consumption at an absolute minimum. As mentioned on page 75, many canned foods contain bisphenol A, which is a hormone disruptor. Some brands are BPA-free, and you may choose to use those canned beans for some recipes.

Sweets

Sweeten your food naturally. For baking, try organic unsweetened applesauce, molasses, real maple syrup, raw honey, yacon syrup, coconut sugar or coconut nectar. For sweetening drinks, try stevia (an herbal sweetener) in liquid or powder form. Some spices naturally sweeten, such as cinnamon, cloves and nutmeg. But don't go crazy with any of these sweeteners. Moderation is key!

Cow's milk alternatives: almond (see recipe on page 170), brown rice, coconut (see recipe on page 168), hemp (see recipe on page 170), quinoa, oat and flaxseed milks

Fancy superfoods (if budget allows): acai powder, camu camu powder, greens powder, goji berries, raw cacao, bee pollen, kombucha, mulberries, maca

Fermented foods: kombucha, kimchi, kefir (provided no sensitivities are present), sauerkraut, miso, tempeh, apple cider vinegar

These foods are high in good bacteria and therefore beneficial for digestion and immunity.

Water

At the bare minimum, a basic carbon filter will remove most of the chlorine and some of the heavy metals from your water. If budget allows, the best choice is a reverse osmosis filter with an attachment that alkalinizes the water. Avoid bottled water and plain tap water if possible. To add more zip to your water, make the limeade on page 168.

Notes on Ingredients

To make your recipes extra joyous, here are some ingredient suggestions.

Baking soda and baking powder: Look for aluminum-free brands. If you want your recipe to be truly gluten-free, make sure it also states this on the label.

Sugars: The most common sugars you will see in my recipes are coconut and Sucanat sugar. Large grocery stores that have a health food section often stock these sugars. They are less refined and contain more nutrients than regular white granular or brown sugar. But remember, at the end of the day sugar is sugar, so use it moderately, as suggested in the recipes.

Choose organic whenever possible for these ingredients:

- All animal foods such as eggs, chicken, turkey, goat cheese
- Dirty Dozen (page 105)
- All fats and oils such as coconut oil, olive oil, butter

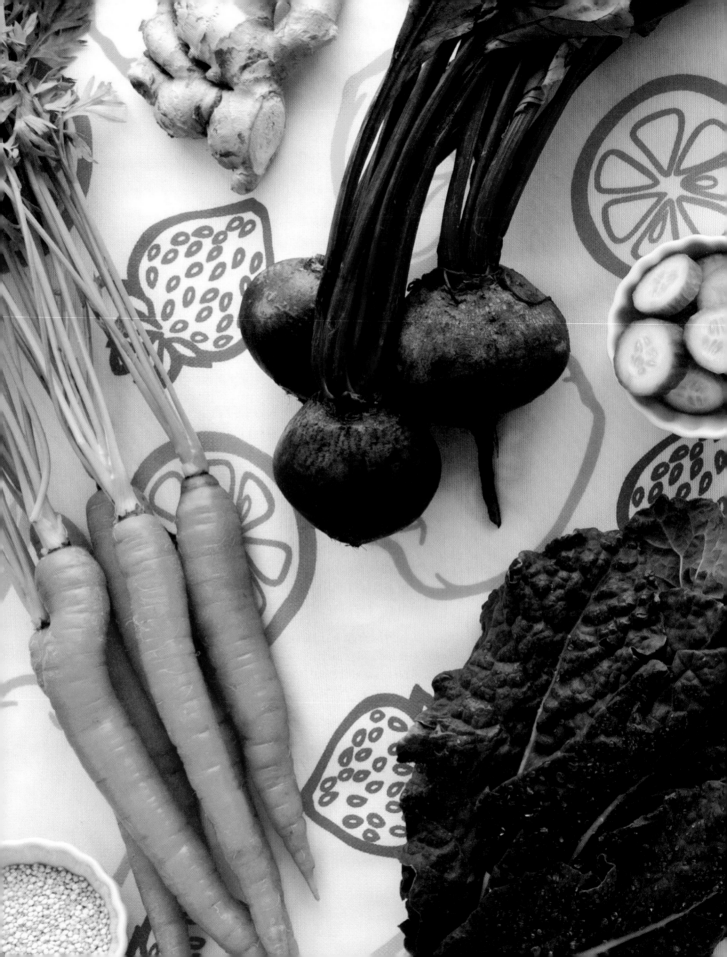

Tips for Joyous Shopping on a Budget

Buying whole, organic foods can make your grocery bill a little higher, but keep in mind that it's better for you and Mama Earth. Here are some tips to help you be a savvy shopper, and you can use the suggested meal plan on page 116.

Write out a weekly menu and a grocery list. Shop according to the meals you are making during the week. This will also help prevent creepy crawlies (i.e., mold) from growing in your fridge. The average North American wastes 40 percent of their groceries because they rot in the fridge! That's not a very joyous thing to do to avocados and kale.

Look for coupons and specials. There are often specials that can be downloaded from a store's website before you go there. Then you can stock up on non-perishable foods or, for example, if your favorite fresh berry is on sale, you can buy extra and freeze them.

Practice Meatless Monday. Organic meat as your main dish costs a heck of a lot more than a vegetarian meal. You will be amazed at how much lower your grocery bills are if you eat more plant-based foods. Start out by choosing one day of the week, such as Monday, to go meatless, meaning no animal foods for the whole day.

Shop seasonally. In-season foods are more nutrient-dense and tastier! Rather than buying hard, flavorless strawberries in the dead of winter, buy them when they are in season. It makes sense to eat this way, just as our ancestors did.

Remember the Dirty Dozen and the Clean 15 (page 105). Several fruits and vegetables are known to have very low pesticide residue, so it's not necessary to purchase these foods organic. As a bonus, you may notice that when a food is in season, the organic version is often the same price as the conventional, sometimes cheaper.

Buy in bulk—it's cheaper. You can purchase grains, pastas, dried fruits, nuts and flours in the bulk aisles of your grocery or natural food store. When fresh fruits or vegetables that can easily be frozen are in season, such as berries, green beans and peas, buy extra and freeze them.

Invest in a Community Supported Agriculture program. These programs allow you to regularly enjoy a share of a local farm's harvest by receiving a weekly box of fresh fruits and vegetables. Not only are you supporting a local farm, but in most cases you're also getting organic produce that's fresher than anything you'll find in a store. Yum!

Brown-bag (or better yet, glass-container) your lunch with leftovers from last night's dinner. I normally cook extra at dinner and eat leftovers for lunch the next day.

Give Your Kitchen a Makeover

Choose one day in the next week or so to do a kitchen makeover. Use this chart as a guide to stocking your kitchen more healthfully.

Instead of This, Eat This: Have a Healthy Substitution

INSTEAD OF THIS …	HAVE A HEALTHIER OPTION!	WHY?
Ketchup	Salsa; hot sauce; chop up avocado, tomato and red onion with lime juice for a quick salsa	Ketchup is mostly refined sugar.
Prepared salad dressing	Combine olive oil and balsamic vinegar, or mix tahini, tamari, fresh ginger, lemon juice (or lemon juice mixed with hemp seed oil and 3 drops stevia). See recipes section for more ideas.	Contains sugar, sodium, preservatives, possibly artificial sweeteners and flavoring agents.
Sauces (e.g., marinades, prepared stir-fry sauces)	Fresh herbs, garlic, spices, Dijon mustard, lemon, balsamic vinegar, tamari	Contain sugar, sodium, flavor enhancers like MSG, additives such as food coloring.
Frozen dinners	Cook on the weekend and freeze leftovers to enjoy throughout the week.	High in sodium; very little nutritional value due to food processing. Excess sugar and additives are often added for flavor.
Cereal bars	Choose loose granola and mix it with dried fruit. Make the Trail Mix on page 215.	Most cereals bars are full of sugar and preservatives with very few "whole" ingredients.
Take-out or frozen pizza	Make your own and top with fresh ingredients on a whole-wheat or gluten-free brown rice crust. Try the pizza recipe on page 246.	Contains trans fats and sodium, high glycemic index (crust high in sugar); nutrient-dead food.
White pasta	Whole wheat, kamut, spelt, buckwheat, brown rice, quinoa. Watch out for spinach pasta. It's just white pasta with spinach or food coloring added for color.	Highly refined food, stripped of B vitamins, essential fatty acids, antioxidants; has little to no fiber. Many synthetic nutrients are added back into white pasta by law. This is why you see B vitamins listed in the ingredients of most white pasta.
Take-out sandwiches/subs	Brown-bag your lunch. Choose a whole-wheat wrap, load it up with veggies and *real* chicken (no luncheon meats), add hummus or avocado.	Fake meats contain nitrates and other food additives. Excess calories from sauces and chemicals.
Flavored canned tuna	Plain tuna or wild salmon—limit to once a week.	Can be high in mercury and sodium; artificial flavoring.
Store-bought muffins, cookies, croissants	Natural almond butter on toast or on apple with cinnamon, homemade muffins	Contains trans fats and excessive amounts of refined sugar; very processed junk food.

INSTEAD OF THIS …	HAVE A HEALTHIER OPTION!	WHY?
Ice cream, frozen yogurt, other frozen treats	Make a dessert smoothie and add ice to make it cold (see pages 162, 164 and 165); make popsicles (pages 257 and 258); freeze grapes or blueberries. You can also make your own ice cream, frozen yogurt and gelato very easily with pure ingredients.	Contain refined sugar and additives such as artificial flavors and colors.
Canned or dehydrated soups	Soups in glass jars	Typically very high in sodium; lack nutritional value; possible BPA contamination.
Hydrogenated peanut butter	Natural nut butters: almond, sunflower, pumpkin, hemp seed	High in sugar; very little nutritional value; often contains trans fat; processed junk food.
Cow's milk	Nut milks: oat, almond, hemp, brown rice	See page 66.
Microwave popcorn	Air-popped or stove-top-popped organic corn with organic butter, sea salt and black pepper	Harmful chemicals in lining of bag (including carcinogenic PFOA); fake butter; mostly GMO corn.
Candy, processed chocolate	Dark, organic fair-trade chocolate	Contains sugar, sodium, preservatives. Dark chocolate is a superfood high in antioxidants.
Liquid oils in plastic containers	Oils in cans or dark glass bottles	Chemicals in plastic can leach into oil; many of these oils are rancid.
French fries	Roasted sweet potatoes	Acrylamide, labeled a "probably human carcinogen," forms naturally during the cooking of fries.
Potato chips	Kale chips (see pages 206 and 208)	Full of salt, preservatives, artificial flavoring and coloring.
Pop	Make the limeade on page 168 or make a fresh juice.	Very high in phosphorus; loaded with sugar.
Orange juice	Choose one of the juice recipes on page 174.	Even though there may be no "added sugar," these juices rapidly spike blood sugar; pasteurization removes all the nutrients.
Mayonnaise	Make your own or use one of the salad dressing recipes on page 193 as a healthy, delicious substitute.	Store-bought mayonnaise is a processed food with many additives.
Margarine	Butter, ghee, olive oil	The plastic of the food industry. I do not consider this a real food. One of the most highly processed foods on the market today.

Joyous Tools for the Kitchen

Stock your kitchen with these tools for the most joyous cooking experience.

Blender

A good-quality blender is very handy in the kitchen because it has such a wide variety of uses, making everything from smoothies, puréed soups and nut butters to hummus and pesto. A broad range is available, from the Mercedes-Benz of blenders—the Vitamix ($500+)—to the budget-friendly Volkswagen—Breville (under $500). I started out with a Breville and have used it for years, but the Vitamix is a pretty sweet machine. The difference between high-end blenders and budget-friendly options is usually the wattage (power) and a few extra bells and whistles. Blending in a Vitamix will be much quicker and more efficient than in some of the less expensive options. Either way, a blender is essential for a joyous, healthy kitchen.

Juicer

Regularly drinking fresh fruit and veggie juices is an amazing way to detoxify the liver and cleanse the colon (otherwise known as beautifying from the inside out)! There are two main types of juicers I recommend: centrifugal juicers and slow upright juicers. There is no one right juicer for everyone because choosing the right juicer depends entirely on your budget and what types of fruits and vegetables you plan on juicing.

Centrifugal juicer: $150 to $350

This is the most budget-friendly juicer and it's perfect for those who do not want to juice lots of leafy greens, wheatgrass or fresh herbs. It's great for foods with a large surface area to juice—apples, pears, beets, celery, carrots and citrus. Keep in mind that the fast-rotating blade that shreds the produce can destroy some of the nutrients, including enzymes. Recommended brand: Breville.

Slow juicer: $350 to $550

This is the most versatile juicer on the market because it will juice any type of produce, from hardest to softest, and any leafy green—hurray! The main difference is that a slow juicer first crushes the food, then presses it to produce the highest juice yield possible while keeping the enzymes and nutrients intact. Bonus: its design takes up much less counter space. Recommended brands: Hurom, Breville.

No matter which juicer you purchase, you will be amazed at how much better fresh juice tastes. Plus, it's higher in naturally occurring nutrients than commercial juice, whose nutrients are added after it's been pasteurized.

Electric Mixer

If you love to bake, then a stand mixer like the KitchenAid ($500+) will seem heaven-sent because it mixes your ingredients so evenly. It's all about wattage when it comes to choosing a good-quality mixer—the more power, the better. Having a variety of speeds, as opposed to just fast and slow, allows you to create a wide range of baked goods just like a pastry chef! Plus it looks pretty on your counter.

If you don't bake a lot, then a hand mixer will do just fine and be far easier on your wallet, at under $100.

Food Processor

Even though a good-quality blender can do many of the jobs of a food processor, the advantage of a food processor is that you can make smaller batches with ease. I suggest a mini food processor (capacity 3 to 4 cups/750 mL to 1 L) for smaller batches of recipes and a large one (7 to 20 cups/1.75 to 5 L) for bigger jobs. I use my mini processor nearly every single day! I love making kale pesto in my mini processor and the Sexy Maca Balls (page 261) in my large one. A mini food processor can cost as little as $40 and a large one can be as much as $1000, though you don't have to spend that much. You can get a decent large food processor for $350 to $500. Recommended brands: Cuisinart, KitchenAid, Breville.

Slicing and Dicing Tools

When I was taking culinary arts courses at George Brown College in Toronto, one of the best pieces of advice I received was to stock your kitchen with really good quality knives and a mandoline. I highly encourage you to make many of the recipes in this book, so having good knives and a mandoline will come in handy. I suggest you use a large wooden cutting board—yet another kitchen essential! Cutting on a glass or marble cutting board can seriously dull your knives. A set of good-quality knives can be found for a good price (a few hundred dollars or less) at Winners. As for a mandoline, you can spend anywhere from $25 to $150.

Food Storage: Glass Containers and Mason Jars

Please, I beg you, *do not* store your food in plastic containers! Even if your plastic is BPA-free, it can still leach chemicals into your food. When you take the time to make good-quality nutrient-dense food, you don't want to ruin it by storing it in plastic. Mason jars are my favorite storage item for liquids such as almond milk or soups. I also love taking them on the go if I make a smoothie for the road. As for storing leftovers, get yourself a package of eight to ten different-sized glass or stainless steel containers with lids. I often see them on sale at hardware stores, so you can get a wide range of sizes for under $30. Stainless steel food containers are kid-friendly because they won't break and are much lighter to carry around.

Joyous Tip

Skip the microwave: Please don't irradiate your food by heating it in a microwave. A study published in the *Journal of the Science of Food and Agriculture* in 2003 found that broccoli microwaved in water lost up to 97 percent of its nutrients, including beneficial flavonoids, some phenolic compounds and glucosinolates. Be sure to eat plenty of raw foods, as any type of cooking leads to some degree of nutrient loss. If you need to heat something, heat it on the stovetop, or heat it in the morning and place it in a thermos that will keep it warm for hours. It will taste far better!

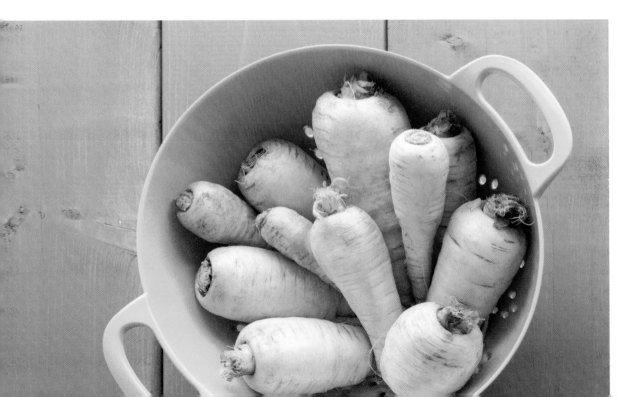

OTHER JOYOUS KITCHEN ESSENTIALS

Nut bag: this makes creating nut milk so much easier and allows you to strain the milk away from the grit with ease.

Citrus zester: for salad dressings and sauces.

Lemon juicer: perfect for your morning water with lemon juice.

Vegetable peeler: you should leave the peel on most fruits and vegetables because that is where most of the nutrients are contained, but a vegetable peeler is great for making thick, flat noodles out of zucchini—a joyous alternative to whole wheat pasta.

Cheese grater (large and small): this comes in handy for shredding cabbage, carrots, beets or even fresh ginger and is a low-budget alternative to a food processor.

Garlic press: I usually chop garlic, but when a recipe calls for minced, it's handy to have a press on hand.

Coffee grinder: very handy for grinding spices and flaxseeds.

Measuring cups and spoons: choose metal, ceramic or glass.

. . .

The right tools are only half the formula for making a meal joyous. Always remember to put love and good intentions into everything you create!

. . .

Colander: a wire colander can replace a nut bag when making nut milk.

Pots and pans: avoid Teflon and other non-stick surfaces because many of these coatings contain carcinogenic chemicals. Choose stainless steel or cast iron (enameled or not) instead.

Grill pan or electric indoor grill: wonderful for a fast, healthy meal of grilled fish or veggies.

Baking dishes: two or three at least, sized from a loaf pan to a lasagna pan. A muffin pan will come in handy too!

Stainless steel, ceramic or glass mixing bowls.

Wooden spoons.

Large and small spatulas.

7

JOYOUS RECIPES

BREAKFAST   136

SMOOTHIES, SIPS
AND JUICES   160

SOUPS   178

SALADS AND SNACKS   192

MAINS AND SIDES   226

DESSERTS   252

. . . .

D Detox

DF Dairy-free

V Vegan
(no animal products)

V Vegetarian
(may include eggs
or dairy)

GF Gluten-free

J Joyous Comfort
(comfort food)

R Raw
(Defined as food not heated above 118°F/48°C.
If you're following a strict raw food diet, look for
raw substitutes for ingredients like tamari sauce
and vanilla extract.)

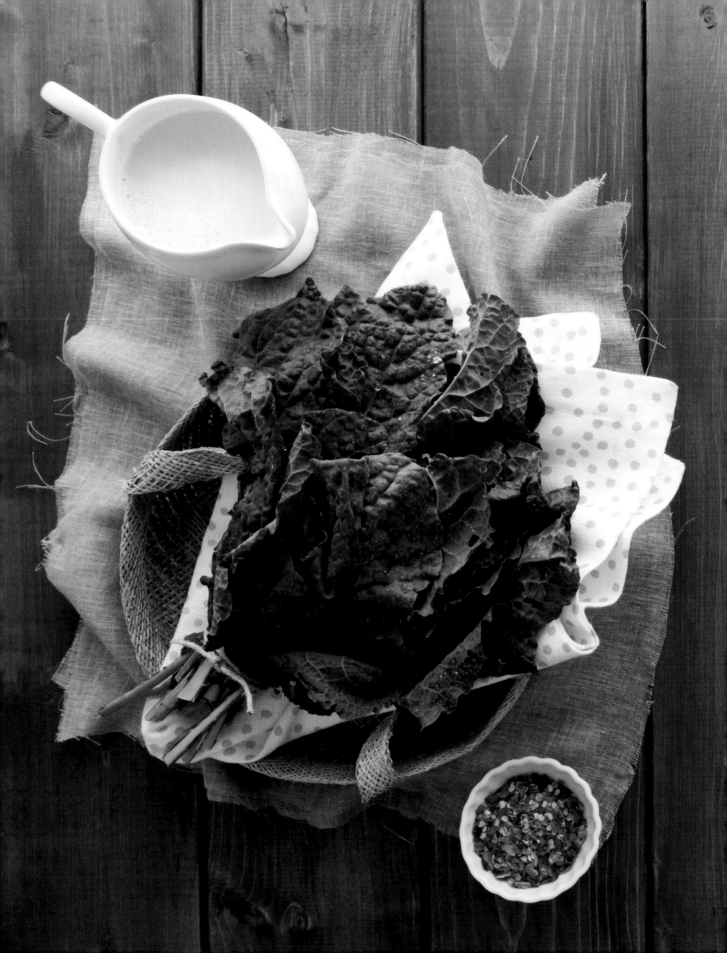

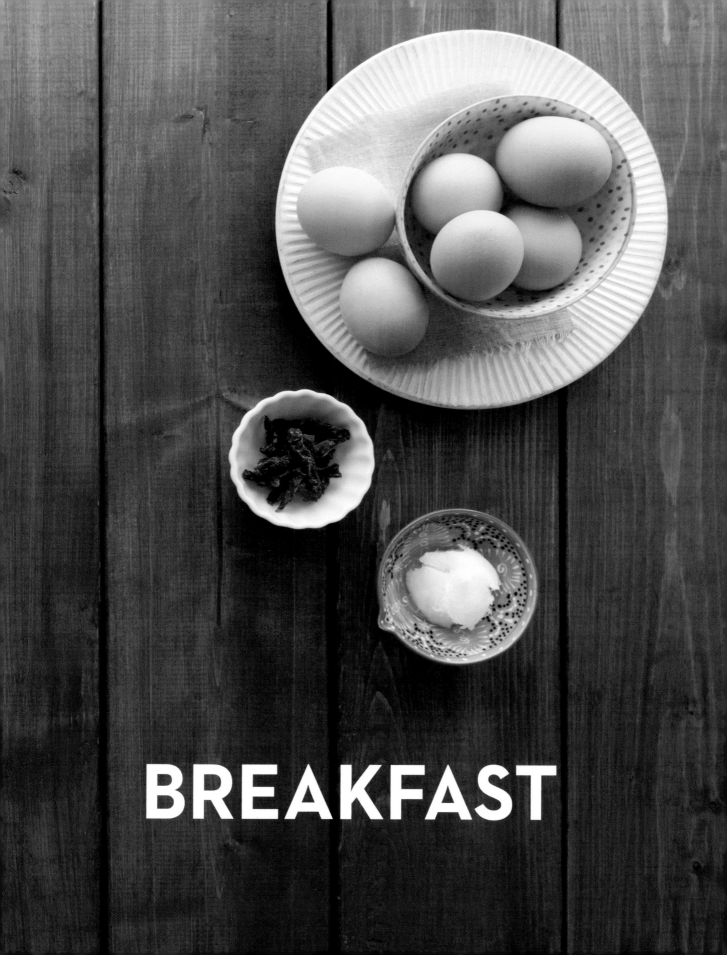

BREAKFAST

Mexican Toast   137

How to Make Perfect Quinoa   137

Apricot Oat Granola Muffins   139

Goji Berry Glory Muffins   140

Quinoa Berry Bowl   142

Apple Walnut Sprouted French Toast   144

Blueberry Spelt Pancakes with Coconut Butter   147

Coconut Flour Banana Pancakes   148

Maple Banana Grilled Sandwich   150

Avocado Kale Tartine   152

Chocolate Protein Squares   154

Overnight Strawberry Chia Pudding   157

Mexican Toast

The flavors in this quick breakfast or snack remind me of my travels in Mexico. I often make a smaller version with brown rice crackers as a mid-afternoon power snack.

Serves 1

 Vegan **DF** **Dairy-free**

2 slices whole-grain or gluten-free bread

1 tsp (5 mL) extra-virgin olive oil

¾ ripe avocado, peeled and sliced

1 small tomato, sliced

¼ cup (60 mL) hemp seeds

Pinch of cayenne pepper

Squirt of lime juice

Toast bread. Drizzle toast with oil. Top with avocado slices, tomato slices and hemp seeds. Sprinkle with cayenne and squirt with lime juice.

How to Make Perfect Quinoa

Many people have told me they have trouble getting their quinoa fluffy and perfectly cooked, so I'm going to tell you exactly how to do it. I always buy pre-washed quinoa because the bitter saponins have already been removed. If your quinoa is not pre-washed, you need to rinse it at least twice before cooking and then once after cooking; otherwise it can be bitter. Some people find even pre-washed quinoa can taste bitter, so rinse it anyway if that is your preference.

Makes about 2½ cups (625 mL)

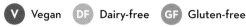 **Vegan** **DF** **Dairy-free** **GF** **Gluten-free**

2 cups (500 mL) filtered water
  (or vegetable or chicken stock for more flavor)

1 cup (250 mL) dry quinoa

In a medium saucepan, bring water and quinoa to a boil. Reduce heat to low, partly cover and simmer, stirring occasionally, for 15 minutes or until quinoa has a fluffy texture and the outer ring has separated from the seed. Remove from heat and fluff with a fork. You can keep quinoa refrigerated in a glass storage container for up to 4 days. Now you're ready for the Quinoa Berry Bowl on page 142.

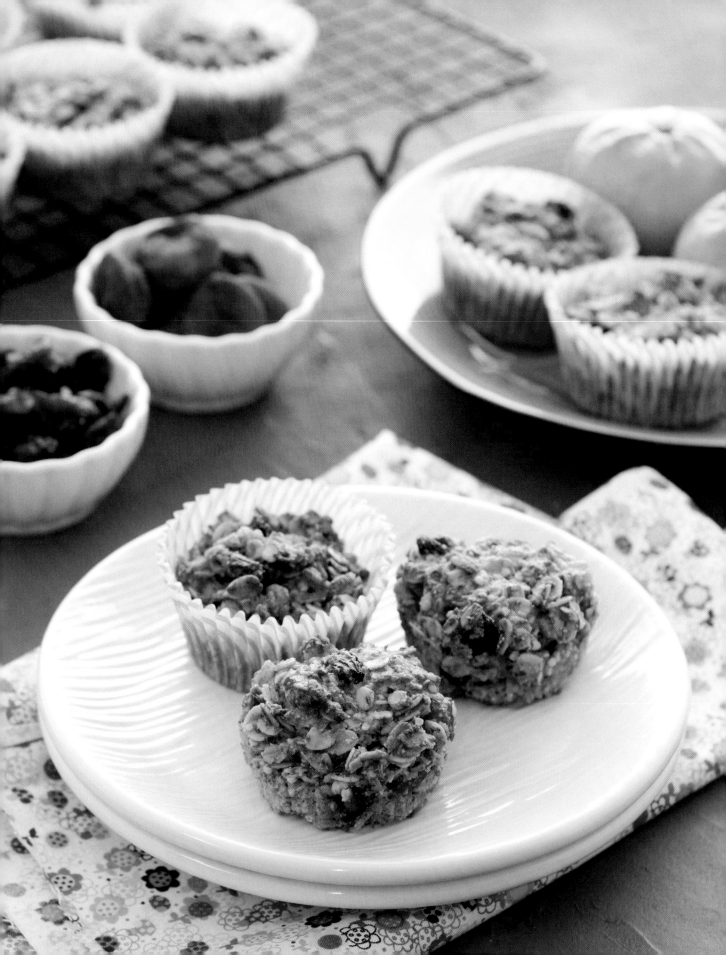

Apricot Oat Granola Muffins

These grab-and-go muffins are perfect for busy mornings when you need something tasty in a hurry. They are hearty enough to fill the hunger gap for a few hours, especially if you slather them with some almond butter.

Makes 12 muffins

V Vegetarian   **DF** Dairy-free

1½ cups (375 mL) quick-cooking rolled oats (not instant)

½ cup (125 mL) almond flour

¼ cup (60 mL) wheat germ

½ cup (125 mL) dried cranberries

½ cup (125 mL) dried apricots, chopped

½ cup (125 mL) pecans or walnuts, chopped

¼ cup (60 mL) sunflower seeds

Grated zest of 2 oranges

1 tsp (5 mL) cinnamon

½ tsp (2 mL) ground ginger

1 large egg

⅔ cup (150 mL) real maple syrup

¼ cup (60 mL) coconut oil, melted

1 tsp (5 mL) pure vanilla extract

Preheat oven to 350°F (180°C). Grease a muffin pan or line with paper liners.

In a large bowl, stir together oats, almond flour, wheat germ, cranberries, apricots, pecans, sunflower seeds, orange zest, cinnamon and ginger. In a separate bowl, lightly beat egg; stir in maple syrup, oil and vanilla. Add wet ingredients to dry ingredients and stir until everything is moist.

Divide batter among muffin cups and pack down tightly with the back of a spoon so they stay together after baking. Bake for 20 minutes or until edges begin to brown. Let cool for several minutes before removing from pan.

Goji Berry Glory Muffins

The spicy sweetness from the cinnamon and ginger will light up your taste buds, and the nourishing ingredients will keep your belly satisfied. I've enjoyed this muffin countless times just before a yoga class. It's just enough to fill the hunger gap, but not too much to weigh you down.

Makes 12 muffins

(V) Vegetarian (DF) Dairy-free (GF) Gluten-free

½ cup (125 mL) goji berries
   (or raisins or dried cranberries)
1 cup (250 mL) brown rice flour
1 cup (250 mL) almond flour
1 cup (250 mL) Sucanat or coconut sugar
2 tsp (10 mL) baking soda
2 tsp (10 mL) cinnamon
½ tsp (2 mL) ground ginger
½ tsp (2 mL) salt
1 apple (unpeeled), cored and finely chopped
2 cups (500 mL) shredded carrots

½ cup (125 mL) unsweetened
   shredded coconut
½ cup (125 mL) chopped walnuts,
   almonds or pecans
⅓ cup (75 mL) pumpkin seeds
3 eggs (any size)
⅔ cup (150 mL) coconut oil, melted,
   or grapeseed oil
¼ cup (60 mL) water or fresh juice
   (orange, apple, pear)
2 tsp (10 mL) pure vanilla extract

Cover goji berries with lukewarm water and let soak for 30 minutes to 1 hour. Drain.

Preheat oven to 350°F (180°C). Grease a muffin pan or line with paper liners.

In a medium bowl, combine rice flour, almond flour, sugar, baking soda, cinnamon, ginger and salt; mix well. In a separate medium bowl, combine goji berries, apple, carrots, coconut, nuts and pumpkin seeds. In a third medium bowl, whisk the eggs with the oil, water and vanilla.

Add egg mixture to fruit and nut mixture; stir well. Add to flour mixture and fold until no dry flour is visible. Do not over-mix.

Divide batter among muffin cups. Bake for 20 to 25 minutes or until golden brown. Let cool slightly before removing from pan.

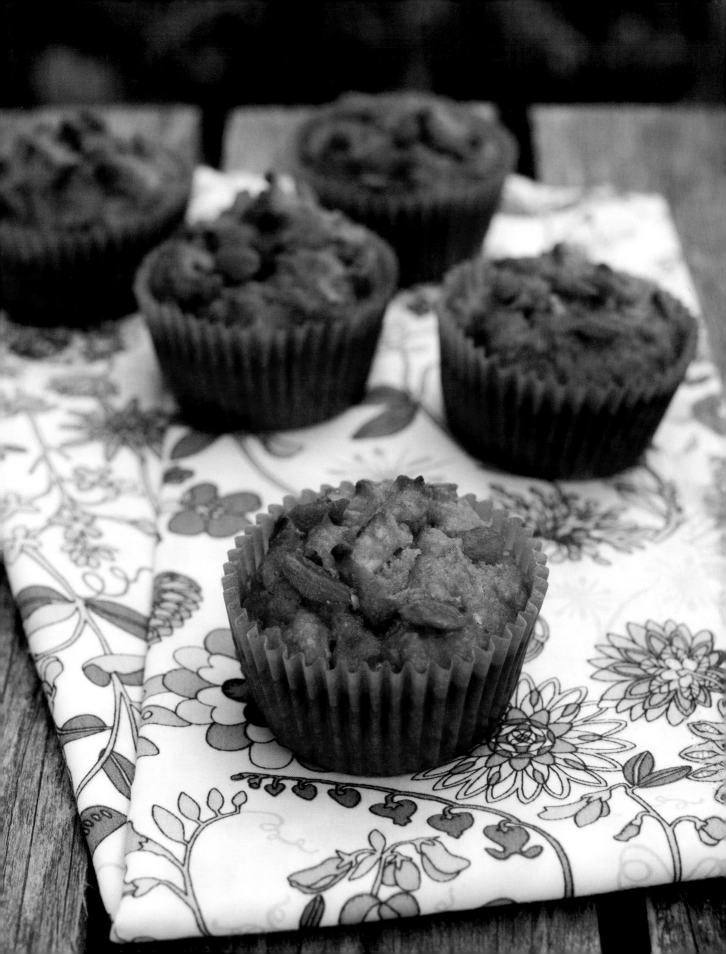

Quinoa Berry Bowl

Ditch the boxed cereals once and for all and indulge in a truly "whole" and "real" breakfast bowl that won't bloat your belly and will keep you completely satisfied for hours thanks to its protein, good fat and fiber. I look forward to this breakfast after a good run or workout. The best thing about this recipe is that you can use whatever ingredients you have on hand, or even better, what's in season! Cook your quinoa ahead of time and breakfast preparation will be even quicker.

Serves 1

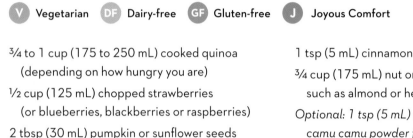 **V** Vegetarian   **DF** Dairy-free   **GF** Gluten-free   **J** Joyous Comfort

¾ to 1 cup (175 to 250 mL) cooked quinoa
    (depending on how hungry you are)
½ cup (125 mL) chopped strawberries
    (or blueberries, blackberries or raspberries)
2 tbsp (30 mL) pumpkin or sunflower seeds
1 tbsp (15 mL) chia seeds
1 tbsp (15 mL) real maple syrup

1 tsp (5 mL) cinnamon
¾ cup (175 mL) nut or seed milk
    such as almond or hemp
Optional: 1 tsp (5 mL) acai or
    camu camu powder for a vitamin C boost

Place quinoa in a cereal bowl and stir in berries, pumpkin seeds, chia seeds, maple syrup, cinnamon and acai, if using. Pour milk on top. Give it a little taste test and add anything else you feel it needs.

. . . .

Joyous Tip

See page 137 for making the perfect quinoa.

. . . .

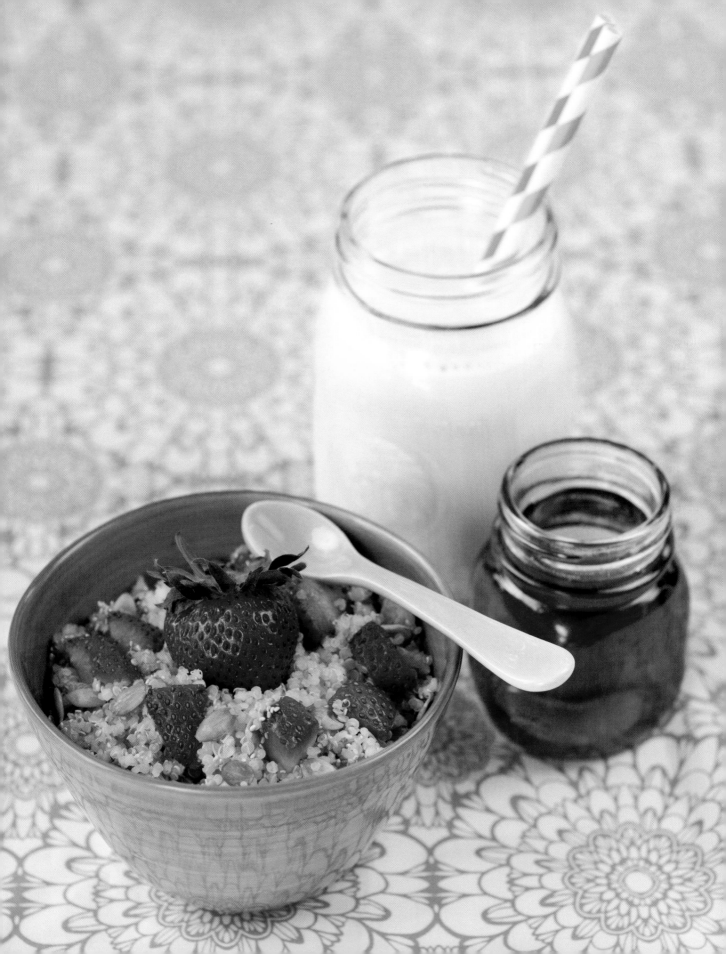

Apple Walnut Sprouted French Toast

Most of the time I don't eat wheat. However, this recipe is an exception because sprouted breads offer a much more digestible form of wheat and are higher in protein. It's become a joyous tradition for me to make this recipe on Sunday mornings for my parents when I visit them at the farm. My nephews and niece call this tradition part of "the Big McCarthy Breakfast."

Serves 4

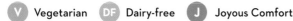 **Vegetarian** **Dairy-free** **Joyous Comfort**

6 eggs

1 cup (250 mL) nut or seed milk
  such as almond or hemp

½ tsp (2 mL) pure vanilla extract

4 tbsp (60 mL) coconut oil

8 slices raisin cinnamon bread
  (I like the Food For Life Ezekiel brand)

½ tsp (2 mL) cinnamon

4 apples (unpeeled), cored and thinly sliced

½ cup (125 mL) walnuts, coarsely chopped

2 tbsp (30 mL) real maple syrup

Preheat oven to lowest setting.

Whisk eggs in a large bowl. Whisk in milk and vanilla.

In a large skillet over medium heat, melt half the coconut oil. Dip 2 or 3 slices of bread into egg mixture, making sure bread is well coated. Place bread in the pan and sprinkle with a little cinnamon. Cook for 4 to 5 minutes. Flip over, sprinkle with cinnamon and cook for another few minutes, until the bottom is golden. Transfer French toast to a baking sheet and keep warm in the oven while you repeat with the remaining bread.

Meanwhile, in another skillet, melt the remaining coconut oil over medium heat. Sauté apples until tender, 5 to 7 minutes. If the pan starts to get dry, add a little more coconut oil. Add walnuts and toss with apples. Remove from heat and drizzle with maple syrup.

Top French toast with sautéed apples. Drizzle with extra maple syrup if you like. Serve immediately.

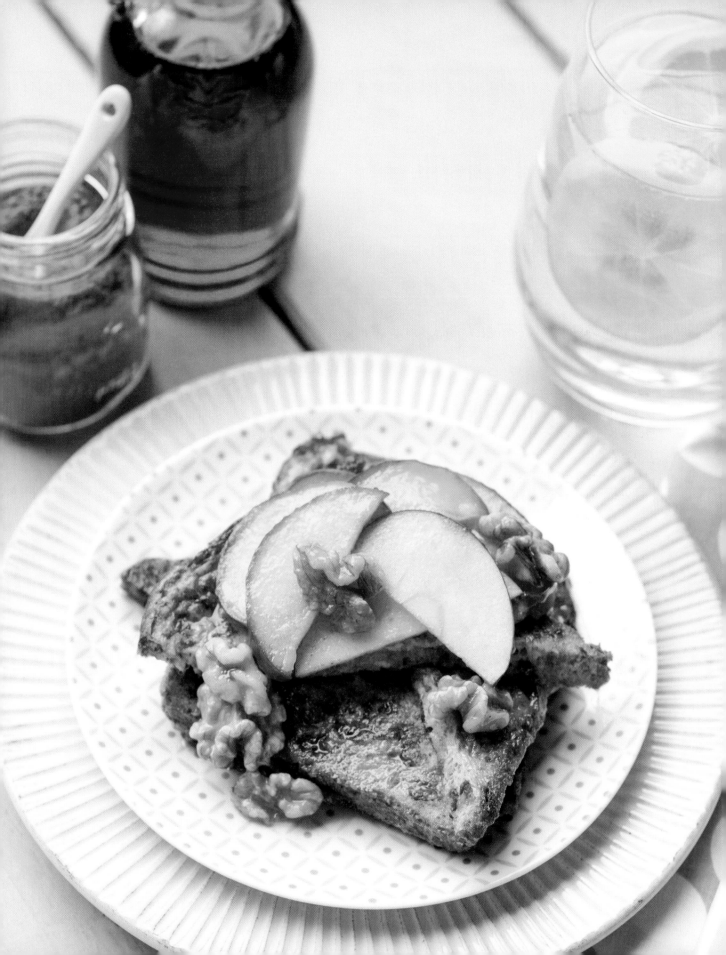

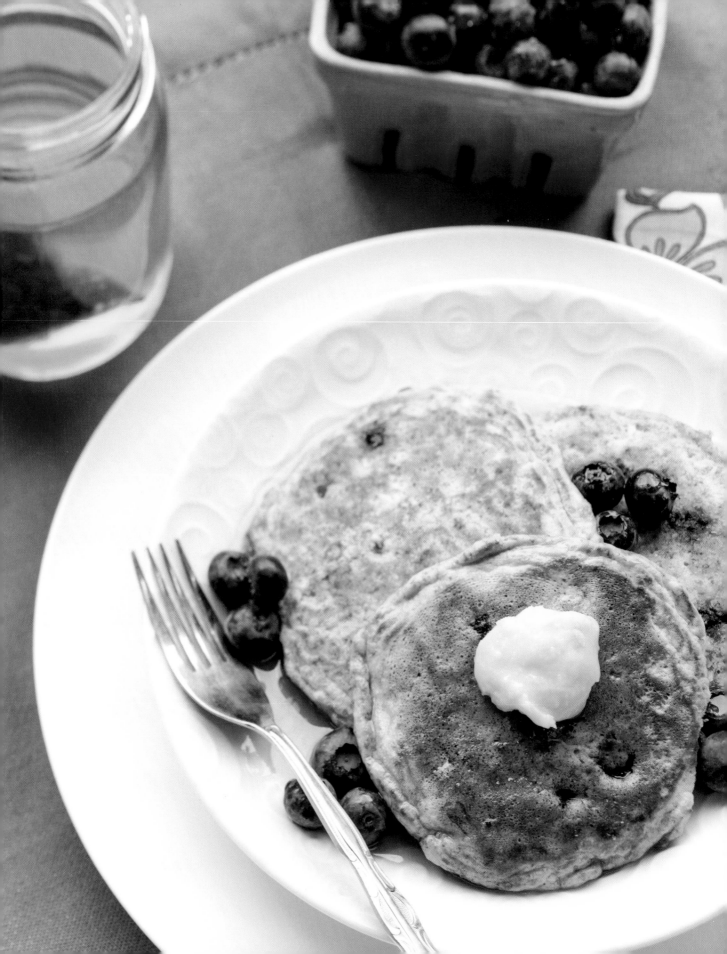

Blueberry Spelt Pancakes with Coconut Butter

This fiber-rich, flavorful breakfast is another "Big McCarthy Breakfast" favorite. Sometimes I make a batch on the weekend, freeze them and then pop them in the toaster during the week—it's like brunch on a weekday in a snap!

Serves 4

(V) Vegetarian   (DF) Dairy-free   (J) Joyous Comfort

1 cup (250 mL) spelt flour

½ cup (125 mL) oat bran

1 tsp (5 mL) baking powder

2 cups (500 mL) almond milk

2 medium eggs, beaten

1 tsp (5 mL) pure vanilla extract

1 cup (250 mL) fresh or frozen wild blueberries

2 tbsp (30 mL) coconut oil

¼ cup (60 mL) coconut butter

In a large bowl, stir together spelt flour, oat bran and baking powder. Add milk, eggs and vanilla; stir until well combined. Fold in blueberries (be sure to thaw and drain excess water if using frozen berries).

Melt coconut oil in a large skillet over medium heat. Pour about ¼ cup (60 mL) batter into the pan for each pancake. Cook for a few minutes, until you see soft bubbles forming on the top and the sides are just turning golden. Flip and cook for a few more minutes, until cooked through. Serve immediately with a dollop of coconut butter. Let it slowly melt on top of your hot pancakes.

. . . .

Joyous Tip

Coconut butter is so naturally sweet you might not even need real maple syrup. My favorite brand is Artisana. Delicious!

. . . .

Coconut Flour Banana Pancakes

These gluten-free pancakes are fluffy and fulfilling. You will be pleasantly surprised to find that they please even the most finicky eaters. Leftovers are fabulous popped in the toaster the next day. You'll feel as if you're having a decadent weekend brunch on a Monday morning.

Makes 6 to 8 pancakes

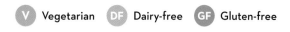 **Vegetarian** **Dairy-free** **Gluten-free**

4 medium eggs, at room temperature

1¼ cups (300 mL) almond milk

1 tsp (5 mL) pure vanilla extract

½ cup (125 mL) coconut flour

1 tsp (5 mL) baking powder

1 tbsp (15 mL) coconut oil

2 bananas, sliced about ¼ inch (5 mm) thick

In a large bowl, whisk eggs. Stir in 1 cup (250 mL) of the milk and vanilla. In a medium bowl, whisk together coconut flour and baking powder.

Add dry ingredients to wet ingredients and whisk just until combined. Some clumps of flour are okay. Let stand for 3 minutes. Lightly whisk again until batter is thick and smooth, similar to brownie batter. Because coconut flour is absorbent, add ¼ cup (60 mL) more almond milk if necessary.

In a large skillet or on a griddle, melt coconut oil over low to medium heat. You may need to add more coconut oil as you go along. Pour about ¼ cup (60 mL) batter into the pan for each pancake. Spread the pancake slightly if your batter is thick. Place 2 or 3 banana slices on top of each pancake. Cook pancakes for a few minutes, until the sides are starting to get golden and the top is forming bubbles. Flip and cook for another 2 to 3 minutes, until cooked through.

. . . .

Joyous Tip

Coconut flour is a great source of fiber—in fact, a mere 2 tbsp (30 mL) has a whopping 6 g of fiber—and it's highly absorbent. This is why eating just two pancakes is very satisfying.

. . . .

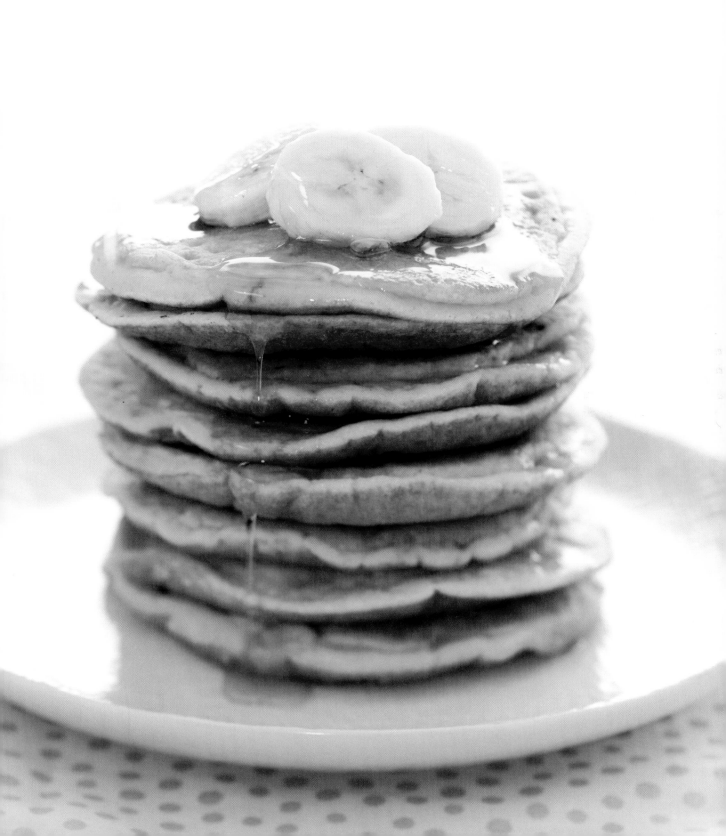

Maple Banana Grilled Sandwich

This grilled sandwich is the breakfast of champions with its protein, complex carbs, good fats, vitamins and minerals. It will keep your belly satisfied until lunch and your brain fueled with lasting energy. It's a hit with kids because they love the natural sweetness from the cinnamon and banana. You could even sneak in a few chia seeds and they won't even know! This sweet breakfast sandwich goes very nicely with a bowl of seasonal fruit.

Serves 1

 V Vegan   **DF** Dairy-free   **J** Joyous Comfort

2 tbsp (30 mL) all-natural sunflower seed butter or almond butter

2 slices sprouted whole wheat bread

1 banana, sliced

1 tsp (5 mL) cinnamon

1 tsp (5 mL) real maple syrup

Optional: 1 tsp (5 mL) chia seeds

Spread sunflower seed butter on one side of each bread slice. Arrange banana slices on top, sprinkle with cinnamon and drizzle with maple syrup. Sprinkle with chia seeds, if using. Top with the other slice of bread, buttered side down.

Heat a grill, skillet or panini press to medium. Cook sandwich, turning once, until golden, 3 to 4 minutes each side.

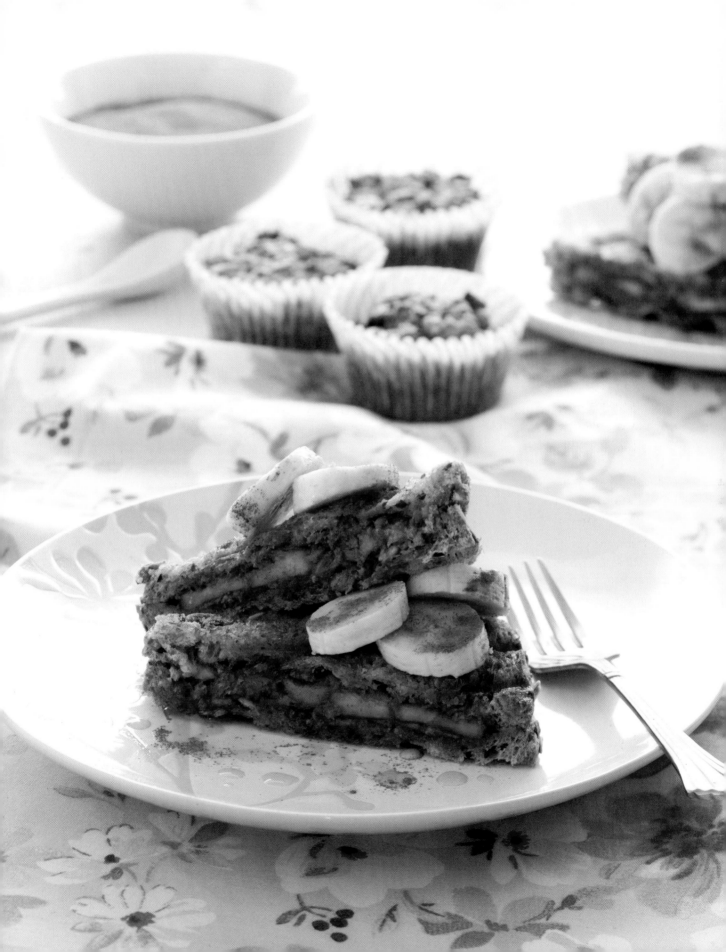

Avocado Kale Tartine

In my opinion, three ingredients that complete a savory breakfast are avocado, kale and eggs. I made this one morning when I was in the mood for something warm and fulfilling. You'll feel like a Parisian with this open-face sandwich!

Serves 1

(V) **Vegetarian**

2 eggs

3 tbsp (45 mL) filtered water

1 tbsp (15 mL) coconut oil

3 kale leaves, washed, stems removed, torn in bite-size pieces

2 slices whole-grain or gluten-free bread

½ ripe avocado, peeled and sliced

A few slices of cucumber and radish or any crunchy vegetables you have on hand for garnish

Sea salt and pepper

1 tbsp (15 mL) extra-virgin olive oil or hemp oil

In a small bowl, whisk eggs with filtered water. Melt coconut oil in a medium skillet over medium heat. Add kale and sauté for a minute. Add eggs and scramble until eggs are completely cooked, 4 to 5 minutes. Remove from heat.

Meanwhile, toast bread.

Place sliced avocado on 1 slice of toast. Top with kale scramble and any crunchy veggies. Season with sea salt and pepper, add a drizzle of oil and garnish as desired. Top with the other slice of toast.

Joyous Tip

Don't be afraid of the whole egg in this recipe. There is a common misconception that the egg yolk is somehow less healthful than the white. This couldn't be further from the truth. In fact, the yolk contains nearly half the protein content of the whole egg and it's a rich source of nutrients, containing far more calcium, vitamin D and folate than the white.

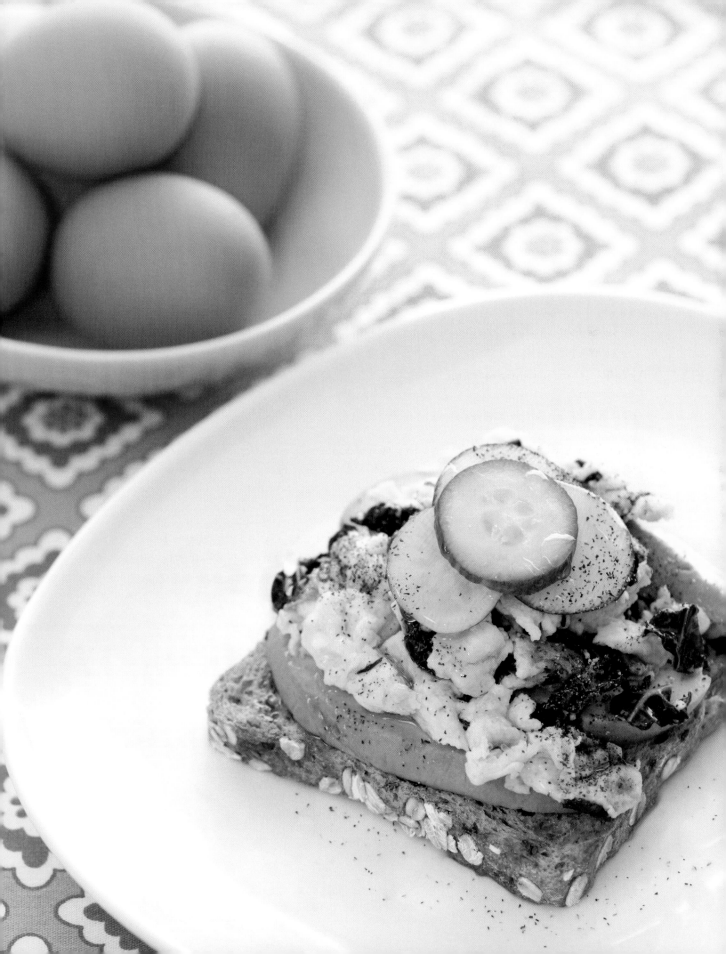

Chocolate Protein Squares

Chocolate for breakfast? Oh yes! These protein-packed squares of deliciousness are the perfect on-the-go breakfast. I often bake them on the weekend and then freeze the individual squares. I simply grab one and head out the door on a busy weekday. They are also lovely as an afternoon crunchy sweet snack. The bars may crumble as you cut them and transfer them to the cookie sheet. Just keep the crumbles and use them as a topping for yogurt—instant homemade granola!

Makes about 20 squares

 Vyan **GF** **Gluten-free**

3 cups (750 mL) raw oats (soaked for 2 hours to increase digestibility) or quick-cooking rolled oats (do not soak)*

1 cup (250 mL) chocolate plant-based protein powder

½ cup (125 mL) sunflower seeds

½ cup (125 mL) unsweetened shredded coconut

½ cup (125 mL) dark chocolate chips or raw cacao nibs

½ cup (125 mL) chopped almonds, walnuts or pecans

¼ cup (60 mL) coconut sugar

1 tsp (5 mL) cinnamon

1 cup (250 mL) almond butter or sunflower seed butter

¼ cup (60 mL) coconut oil

½ cup (125 mL) almond milk

2 tbsp (30 mL) real maple syrup

1 tsp (5 mL) pure vanilla extract

This recipe is gluten-free only if you use oats labeled "gluten-free." Oats can be contaminated with wheat.

Preheat oven to 350°F (180°C). Grease a 13×9-inch (3 L) baking dish.

In a large bowl, combine oats, protein powder, sunflower seeds, coconut, chocolate chips, almonds, sugar and cinnamon; mix well.

In a small saucepan over low heat, melt almond butter and coconut oil. Add to dry ingredients; add almond milk, maple syrup and vanilla. Stir until fully combined. Give it a little taste test, adding more maple syrup if you desire a sweeter taste.

Pour batter into the baking dish and press it down evenly with wet hands. Bake for 15 minutes. Remove from oven and let cool slightly. Cut bars into your desired size and transfer them to a greased cookie sheet. Bake for another 10 to 12 minutes or until the edges are golden brown. Let cool for a few minutes on the baking sheet. Serve immediately or transfer to a rack to cool completely. Store in an airtight container for a week or freeze for a few months.

Joyous Tip

Have you ever read the ingredients on a package of protein or energy bars and scratched your head in confusion? I'm not surprised. There are more ingredients in many store-bought bars than in a bag of candy, and that's a lot!

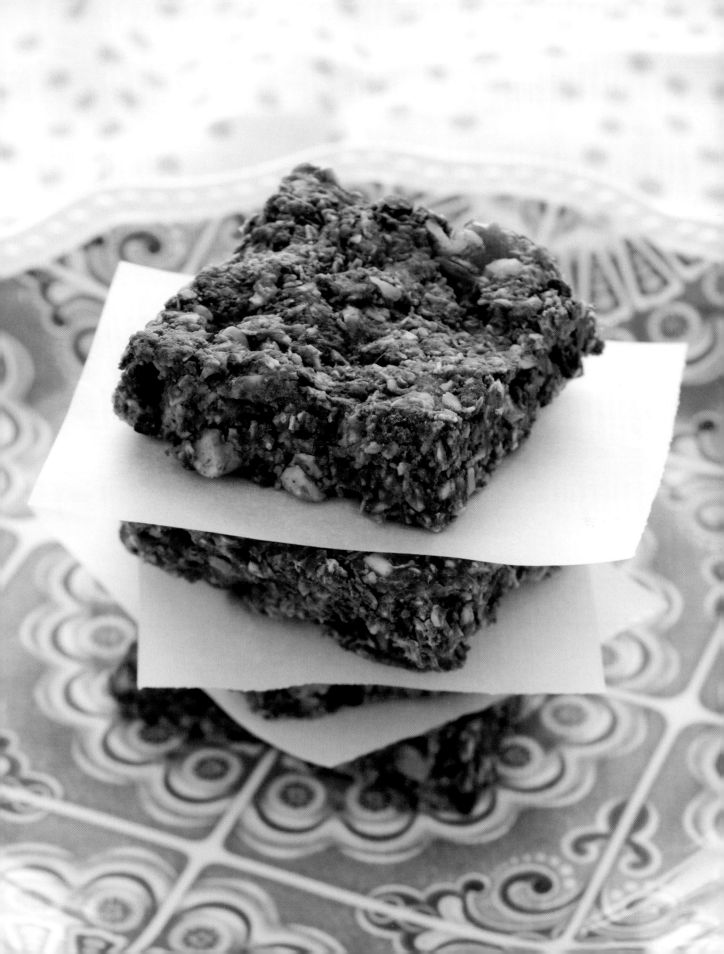

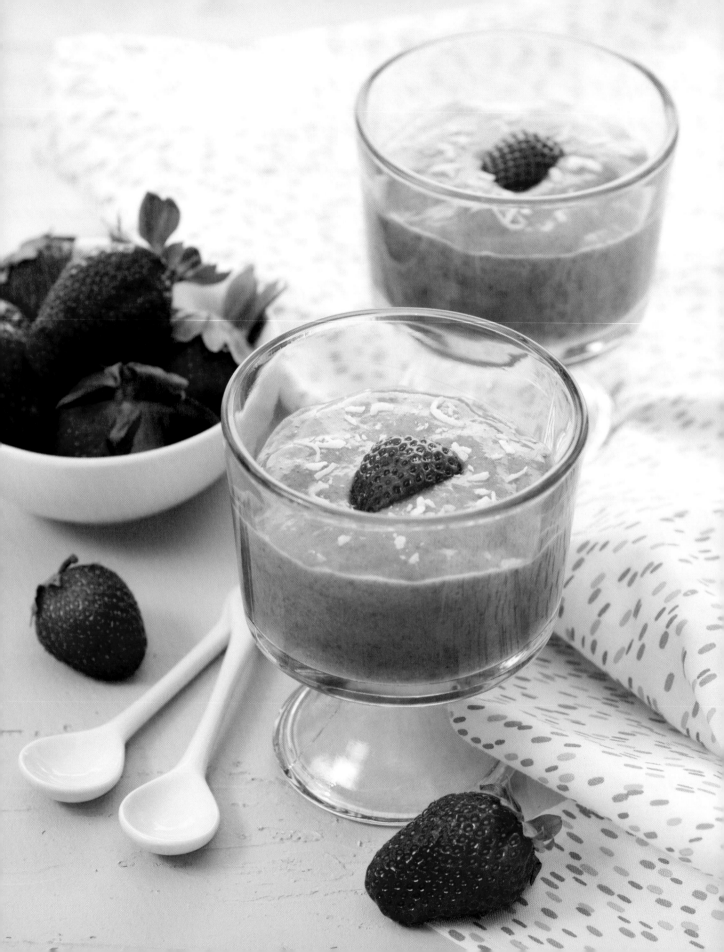

Overnight Strawberry Chia Pudding

Dessert for breakfast, but healthy of course! This wonderfully simple recipe is ideal for those who are dairy-intolerant because you won't miss yogurt one bit. The chia seeds add protein and fiber, while the banana and strawberries make it naturally sweet. It's so yummy you could also enjoy it as a dessert.

Serves 4 to 6

D Detox **V** Vegan **DF** Dairy-free **GF** Gluten-free **J** Joyous Comfort

1 banana

2½ cups (625 mL) fresh or frozen strawberries

1 cup (250 mL) coconut milk or almond milk

¾ cup (175 mL) chia seeds

1 tsp (5 mL) pure vanilla extract

Chopped fresh strawberries for garnish

In a food processor, combine banana, strawberries, coconut milk, chia seeds and vanilla. Process until completely combined. Transfer to a bowl, cover and refrigerate overnight. Divide among bowls and top with chopped strawberries.

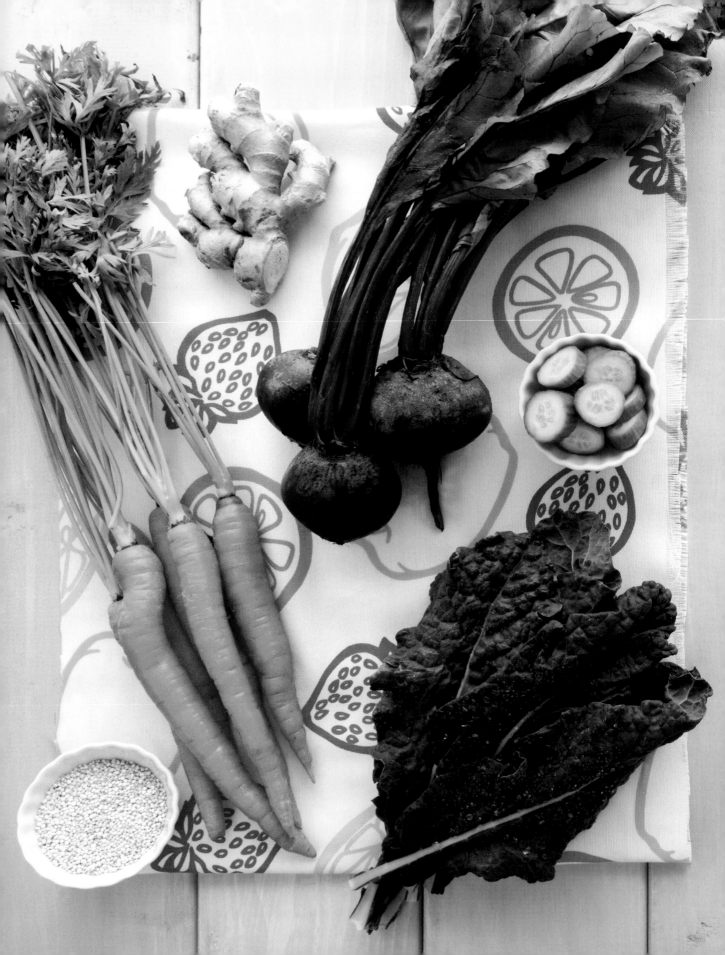

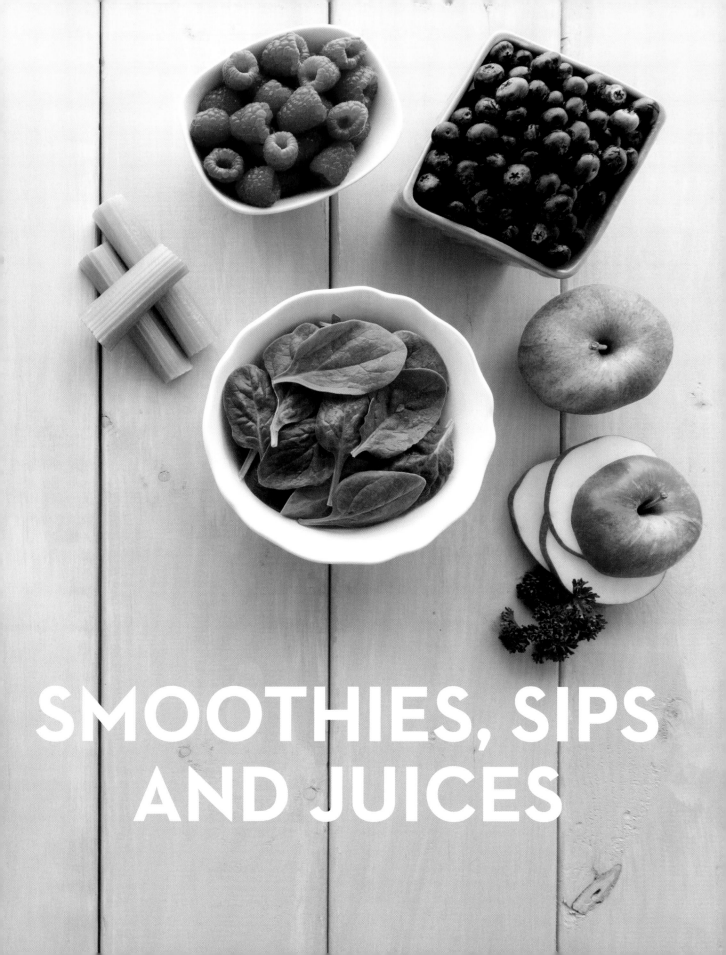

SMOOTHIES, SIPS AND JUICES

Raspberry Chocolate Cheesecake Smoothie   162

Green Goddess Smoothie   164

Morning Energizer Blueberry Smoothie   165

Sangria Kombucha   166

Limeade with Fresh Mint   168

Rich and Fulfilling Coconut Milk   168

Vanilla Almond Milk   170

Creamy Hemp Milk   170

Sunshine Juice   174

Green Beauty Juice   174

Detox Juice   174

Why I Love Smoothies

NUTRIENT-DENSE:
Smoothies are a convenient way for you to get a whole bunch of nutrients in a single meal. Super-easy to make, they can easily be taken on the go, which is much better than skipping a meal altogether.

SOURCE OF PROTEIN:
Protein is an essential component of a joyous smoothie. It keeps cravings away, balances blood sugar, boosts metabolic rate, enhances detoxification and is important for the production of hormones, antibodies and enzymes. My favorite powder brands for a hit of protein are Sunwarrior, because it's made with a highly digestible sprouted brown rice protein, and Genuine Health's Vegan Proteins+ blend. You can also get added protein from some superfoods such as hemp, quinoa and chia.

EASY WAY TO GET SUPERFOODS IN YOUR BEAUTIFUL BODY:
You can add any superfood to your smoothie: bee products, hemp seeds, maca, spirulina, raw cacao, avocado, chia seeds, leafy greens, berries, acai berries, coconut oil or any other ingredient mentioned in the superfoods section (see page 90). These foods contain high levels of beneficial antioxidants, vitamins and minerals.

Raspberry Chocolate Cheesecake Smoothie

This smoothie is so decadent, you'll fool yourself into thinking it's a guilty pleasure. But it's full of goodness, making it completely guilt-free.

Makes 1 or 2 smoothies

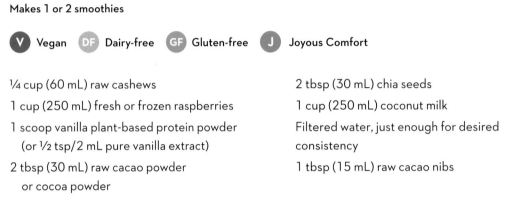 **Vegan**   **DF** Dairy-free   **GF** Gluten-free   **J** Joyous Comfort

¼ cup (60 mL) raw cashews

1 cup (250 mL) fresh or frozen raspberries

1 scoop vanilla plant-based protein powder (or ½ tsp/2 mL pure vanilla extract)

2 tbsp (30 mL) raw cacao powder or cocoa powder

2 tbsp (30 mL) chia seeds

1 cup (250 mL) coconut milk

Filtered water, just enough for desired consistency

1 tbsp (15 mL) raw cacao nibs

Soak cashews in filtered water for about 30 minutes to 1 hour; drain. Place all ingredients except cacao nibs in a blender. Blend for 30 to 60 seconds, until smooth. Pour into a glass and sprinkle with cacao nibs for a nice crunch.

. . . .

Joyous Tip

If your raspberries are a bit tart, add 8 to 10 drops of liquid stevia to sweeten the smoothie.

. . . .

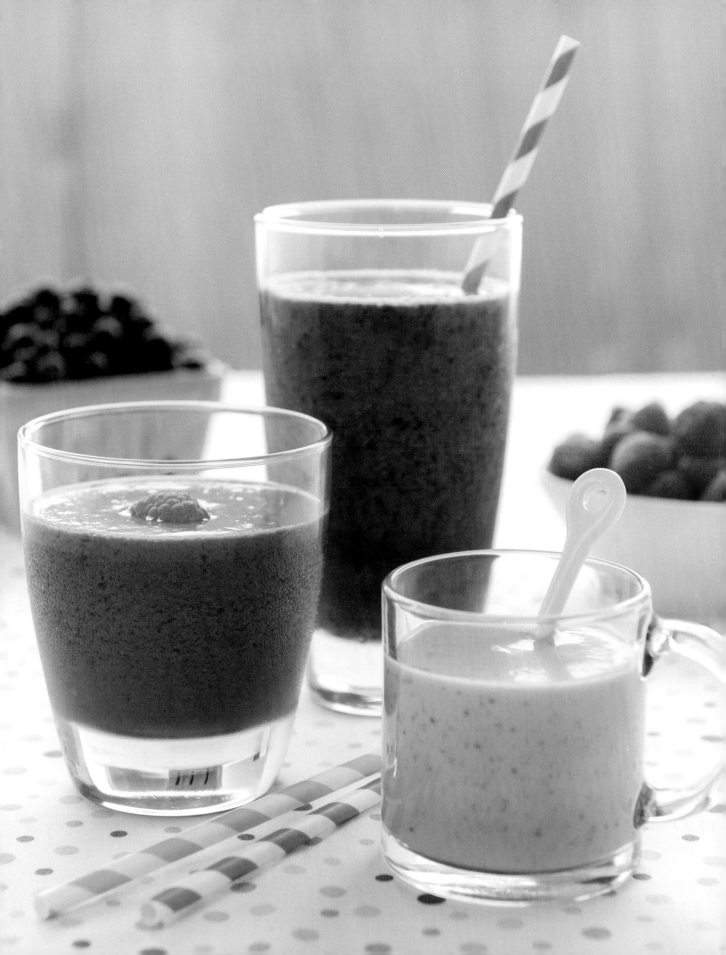

Green Goddess Smoothie

This smoothie is a match made in nutrition heaven because the plant-based protein and good fat will keep your belly full for hours. And the green ingredients, including spinach, kale and mint, are a good source of detoxifying chlorophyll and fiber. Bonus: it's super yummy!

Makes 1 or 2 smoothies

D Detox **V** Vegan **DF** Dairy-free **GF** Gluten-free

2 tbsp (30 mL) hemp seeds

1 banana

½ ripe avocado, peeled

1 cup (250 mL) spinach

1 cup (250 mL) frozen tropical fruit
  (pineapple or mango)

½ cup (125 mL) kale torn in large pieces,
  stems removed

2 tbsp (30 mL) chia seeds

¼ tsp (1 mL) chopped fresh mint

1 cup (250 mL) almond or hemp milk

Filtered water, just enough for desired
  consistency

Reserve 1 tbsp (15 mL) hemp seeds for garnish. Place all ingredients in a blender. Blend for 30 to 60 seconds, until smooth. Pour into a glass and garnish with reserved hemp seeds.

Morning Energizer Blueberry Smoothie

This is a meal in a cup! I always feel balanced and energized for the day when I start my morning off with this smoothie. When blueberries are not in season, I just swap for a different berry or use frozen berries.

Makes 1 or 2 smoothies

 Detox **V** **Vegan** **DF** **Dairy-free** **GF** **Gluten-free**

1 banana

1 cup (250 mL) blueberries

1 cup (250 mL) spinach

¼ cup (60 mL) cooked quinoa

2 tbsp (30 mL) chia seeds

2 tbsp (30 mL) liquid honey*

1 tbsp (15 mL) bee pollen*

1 cup (250 mL) almond milk or hemp milk

Filtered water, just enough for desired consistency

Place all ingredients in a blender. Blend for 30 to 60 seconds, until smooth. Pour into a glass.

If you have any allergies to bees, don't add the bee pollen or honey. Replace the bee product with an equal amount of real maple syrup.

. . . .

Joyous Tip

If you don't have cooked quinoa on hand, add 1 scoop of your favorite plant-based protein powder.

. . . .

Sangria Kombucha

I love entertaining guests. When I do, I always make this sangria kombucha. Luckily, a girlfriend of mine is the creator of my favorite brand, Tonica Kombucha, a beverage full of good bacteria to make your digestive system joyous. This jug is full of so many amazing flavors and bright colors. I'm sure you'll love it!

Serves 6 to 8

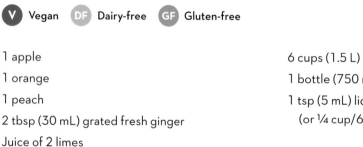 Vegan   Dairy-free   Gluten-free

1 apple

1 orange

1 peach

2 tbsp (30 mL) grated fresh ginger

Juice of 2 limes

6 cups (1.5 L) plain kombucha

1 bottle (750 mL) your favorite red wine

1 tsp (5 mL) liquid stevia
  (or ¼ cup/60 mL liquid honey)

Chop the fruit into large chunks, discarding cores, seeds and pits. Combine all ingredients in a large jug.

Joyous Tip

Prefer a non-alcoholic option? Swap the red wine for cranberry, blueberry or pomegranate juice. These juices are chock-full of antioxidants thanks to their rich colors.

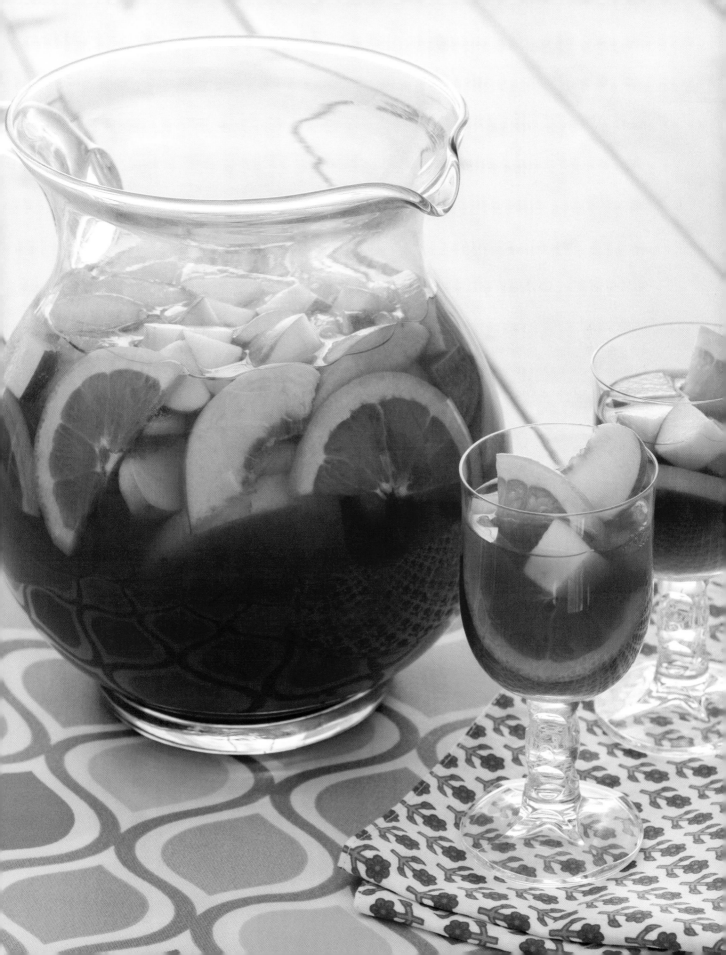

Limeade with Fresh Mint

This thirst-quenching drink will hydrate you from the inside out. A well-hydrated body will be reflected in your skin's health. This limeade is an easy way to ensure you get enough water—and it is incredibly refreshing.

Serves 1

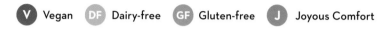 **V** Vegan   **DF** Dairy-free   **GF** Gluten-free   **J** Joyous Comfort

Juice of 2 limes

3 to 5 drops liquid stevia (depending how sweet you like it)

2 tbsp (30 mL) finely chopped fresh mint

1½ cups (375 mL) chilled filtered water

Combine all ingredients in a large glass. Quadruple the recipe if you want to make a jug.

Rich and Fulfilling Coconut Milk

Makes about 4 cups (1 L)

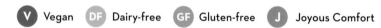 **V** Vegan   **DF** Dairy-free   **GF** Gluten-free   **J** Joyous Comfort

2 cups (500 mL) unsweetened flaked or shredded coconut

4 cups (1 L) filtered water

½ tsp (2 mL) pure vanilla extract

Soak coconut in water for 2 to 4 hours; drain. Place coconut, filtered water and vanilla in a blender. Blend for 60 seconds. Strain through a fine-mesh sieve or a nut bag set over a bowl. Press down on the coconut mixture to release all of the milk. Coconut milk keeps in the fridge for up to 5 days.

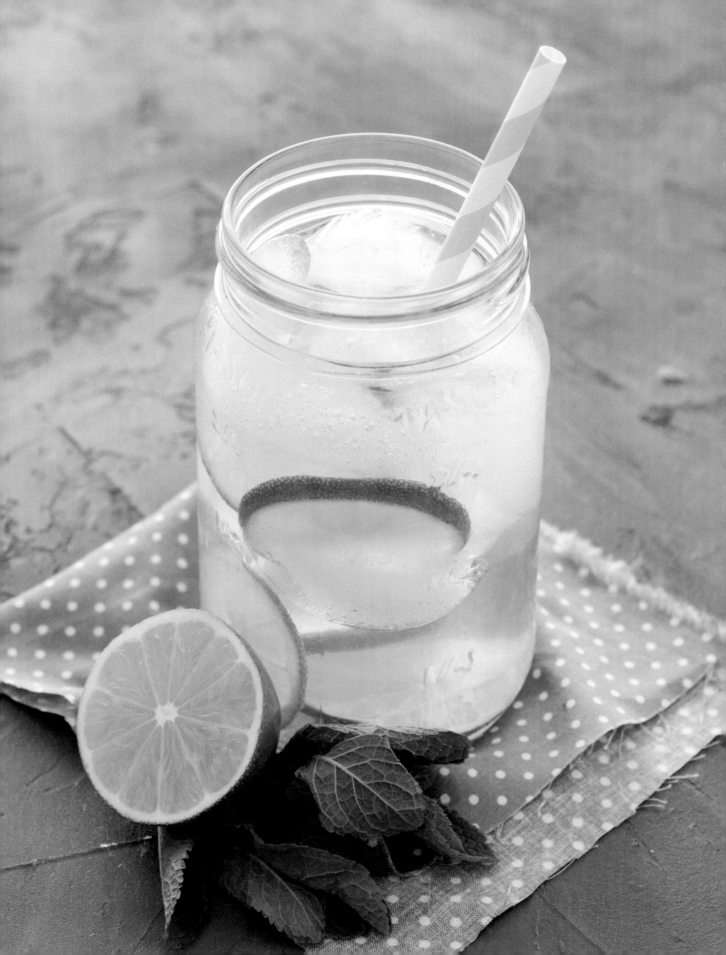

Vanilla Almond Milk

Once you start making your own almond milk rather than buying it, you'll be hooked! You'll never want to buy store-bought again. The taste tells all. Even better, you can easily avoid some nasty additives such as carrageenan. Enjoy in a smoothie or with porridge or granola. Use in place of cow's milk.

Makes about 4 cups (1 L)

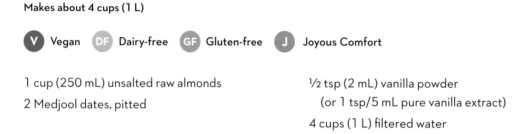

(V) Vegan　(DF) Dairy-free　(GF) Gluten-free　(J) Joyous Comfort

1 cup (250 mL) unsalted raw almonds

2 Medjool dates, pitted

½ tsp (2 mL) vanilla powder
  (or 1 tsp/5 mL pure vanilla extract)

4 cups (1 L) filtered water

Soak almonds in plenty of water overnight. Drain and rinse well.

In a blender, combine almonds, dates, vanilla and water. Blend for 30 to 60 seconds, until you can no longer see any almond chunks. Strain through a fine-mesh sieve or nut bag set over a bowl. Press down on the almond mixture to release all of the milk. It's that easy! Almond milk keeps in the fridge for up to 5 days.

Creamy Hemp Milk

Hemp seeds are a superfood, full of good fat, especially anti-inflammatory GLA. Hemp milk makes a nice change from almond milk. This recipe is incredibly easy!

Makes about 4 cups (1 L)

(V) Vegan　(DF) Dairy-free　(GF) Gluten-free　(J) Joyous Comfort

1 cup (250 mL) hemp seeds

4 cups (1 L) filtered water

Place hemp seeds and water in a blender. Blend well. Strain through a fine-mesh sieve or nut bag set over a bowl. Press down on the hemp mixture to release all of the milk. Hemp milk keeps in the fridge for up to 5 days.

Yummy hemp milk variations:

Add ½ tsp (2 mL) grated orange zest

Add 2 tbsp (30 mL) raw cacao powder

Add ½ tsp (2 mL) cinnamon, cardamom or nutmeg

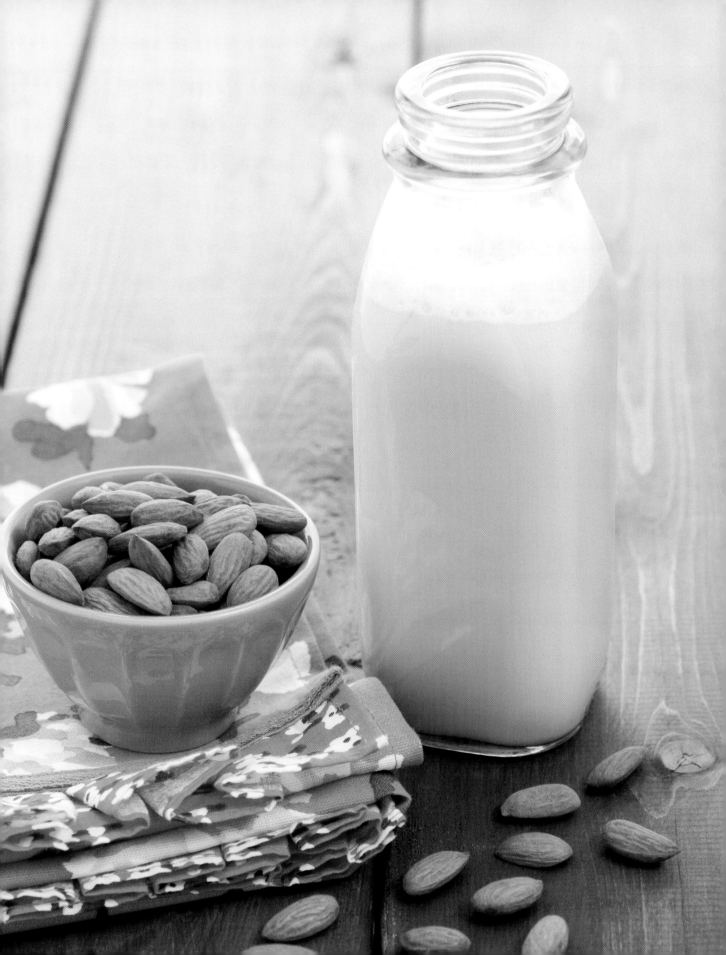

Why I Love Juicing

DETOXIFYING:
Nutrients in many fruits and vegetables, especially brightly colored ones such as beets, carrots, apples, kale, collards and Swiss chard, stimulate the liver's detoxifying pathways to enhance the body's ability to remove toxins.

BONE-BUILDING:
Green vegetables in particular provide a mega-dose of minerals, including calcium, magnesium, iron, potassium and chromium.

BEAUTIFICATION:
Vegetables are high in vitamin C. Just 1 cup (250 mL) of kale provides 70 percent of our recommended daily intake of vitamin C with only 20 calories. Vitamin C is a precursor to collagen, a skin protein responsible for preventing premature wrinkles.

ALKALINIZING:
We could all use more alkalinizing foods in our diet. Most people's bodies are very acidic because of stress, sugar, caffeine, red meat, processed foods and a lack of exercise (or too much exercise). Plant foods are alkaline, making them helpful in balancing your body's pH level.

NUTRIENT-DENSE:
Juicing provides the body with a mega-dose of enzymes (because you are using all raw produce), vitamins, minerals and antioxidants. Scientists are discovering new plant medicines all the time, so there are literally hundreds of beneficial compounds in every cup of juice.

Joyous Tips for Juicing

ALWAYS JUICE 80 PERCENT VEGETABLES AND 20 PERCENT FRUIT.
This will ensure your juice is low on the glycemic index (meaning you won't have a blood sugar spike, keeping your insulin levels in check). This ratio also helps prevent weight gain in the long term.

DOUBLE-JUICE YOUR INGREDIENTS TO GET MORE BANG FOR YOUR BUCK.
You'll get more juice out of your fruits and veggies if you run them through your juicer twice. Bonus: it results in less waste. However, some juicers are so efficient that the pulp is nearly dry and you can skip this step.

USE THE LEFTOVER PULP TO MAKE SOUP STOCK, OR COMPOST IT.
If you plan on using the pulp to make a vegetable stock, make sure you remove any seeds. Some fruit seeds—such as apple—contain naturally occurring toxic substances.

CHOOSE ORGANIC.
When you juice, you concentrate the pesticides because you're actually juicing more of the ingredient than you'd normally eat. Choose organic as often as possible, especially for the "Dirty Dozen" (see page 105).

USE INGREDIENTS THAT ARE IN SEASON.
They'll be the most nutrient-dense, as they've probably been picked ripe and haven't traveled thousands of miles to get to your grocery store. Plus, they are likely cheaper than fruits and vegetables from far away.

BEST INGREDIENTS FOR JUICING:
Cucumbers, celery, Swiss chard and spinach combined with either an apple or a pear. Fresh ginger adds a wonderful uplifting flavor. Herbs such as mint or parsley can also be juiced—both are very refreshing. There are so many choices when it comes to juicing—the only limitation is your creativity!

LASTLY, REMEMBER THAT A FRESH JUICE DOES NOT REPLACE A MEAL.
The best time to drink a fresh juice is first thing in the morning on an empty stomach, or in the middle of the afternoon, again preferably on an empty stomach, as a way to re-energize.

Joyous Juices

Each recipe makes 1 to 2 cups (250 to 500 mL)

 Detox   **V** Vegan   Dairy-free   **GF** Gluten-free   **R** Raw

Sunshine Juice

This juice is an immune-booster with the nutrients in the carrots, ginger, lemon and orange, including beta-carotene and vitamin C. Plus the lemon is incredibly alkalinizing and liver detoxifying. This tastes like sunshine in a cup!

3 carrots

½ cucumber

1 thumb-size piece fresh ginger

1 lemon, peeled and seeded

1 orange or grapefruit, peeled

Cut vegetables and fruits into large chunks depending on the size of the mouth of your juicer. You may run ¼ cup (60 mL) filtered water through the juicer at the end to get every last drop of juice.

Green Beauty Juice

This juice is beautifying because it is extremely hydrating, detoxifying and nutrient-dense. The mint gives it a refreshing lift!

½ cucumber

4 stalks celery

1 apple or pear

3 kale leaves

2 cups (500 mL) spinach

½ cup (125 mL) fresh mint leaves

Cut vegetables and fruits into large chunks depending on the size of the mouth of your juicer. Make sure you remove the seeds from the apple or pear. You may run ¼ cup (60 mL) filtered water through the juicer at the end to get every last drop of juice.

Detox Juice

Get ready to love your liver with this juice featuring beets, carrots and apple. It's also very immune-building. The beet greens can be juiced as well. They can be bitter, but any bitter taste is good for digestion.

3 beets

3 carrots

½ cucumber

1 apple

1 lemon, peeled

1 thumb-size piece fresh ginger

Cut vegetables and fruits into large chunks depending on the size of the mouth of your juicer. Make sure you remove the seeds from the apple and lemon. You may run ¼ cup (60 mL) filtered water through the juicer at the end to get every last drop of juice.

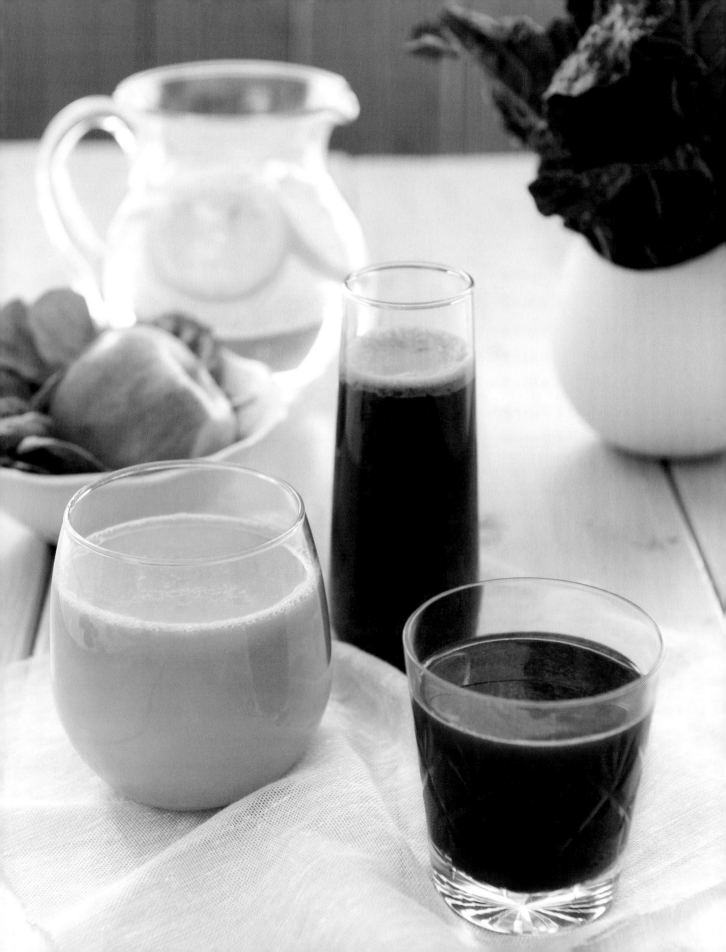

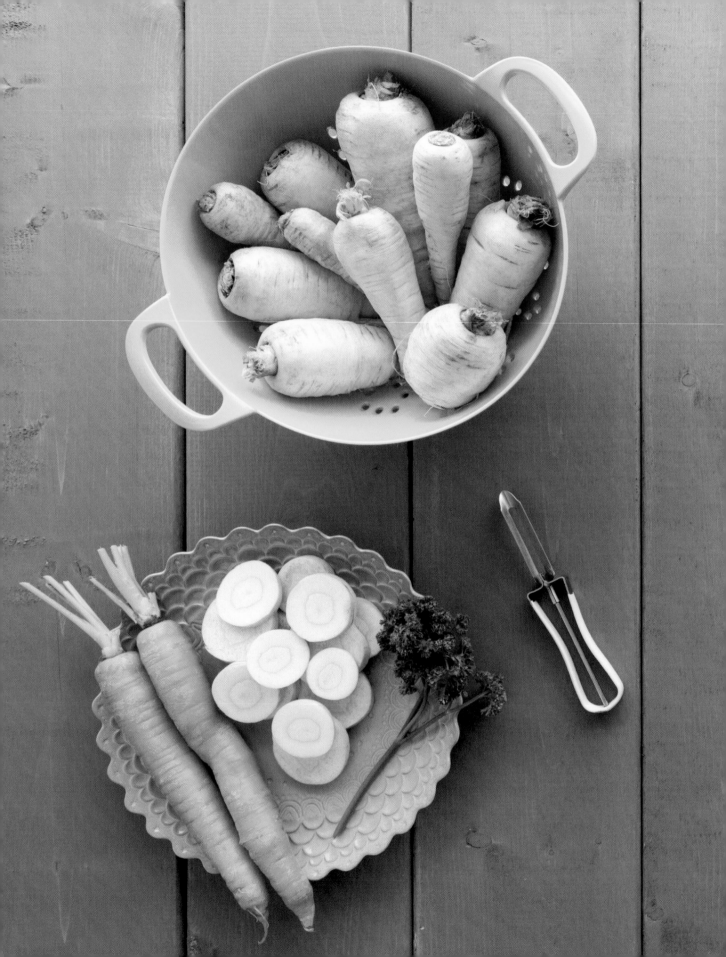

SOUPS

Ma McCarthy's Chicken Soup   179

Carrot Ginger Soup with Lemon Tahini Drizzle   180

Chilled Cucumber Avocado Soup   182

Chicken or Turkey Stock   182

Summer Lovin' Gazpacho   184

Cardamom Parsnip Pear Soup   186

Mama Bea's Curry Lentil Soup   188

Thai Beet Soup   189

Ma McCarthy's Chicken Soup

Ever since I was a little girl, my mom's chicken soup has been a cure-all. Lucky for me, I still get a Mason jar or two to take back home after visiting my parents for the weekend. When I asked my mom for her recipe, she said, "I just make it from scratch off the top of my head every time." I finally persuaded her to write down her secret recipe for me to share! Garlic isn't in the original, but I sometimes add it, as it's an incredible immunity builder.

Serves 8 to 10

 DF Dairy-free **J** Joyous Comfort

16 cups (3.8 L) chicken stock (page 182 or organic low-sodium store-bought)

2 cans (28 oz/796 mL each) diced tomatoes (or 6 to 8 medium tomatoes)

2 tbsp (30 mL) coconut oil or grapeseed oil

1 medium onion, cut in bite-size pieces

2 cloves garlic, minced

2 cups (500 mL) carrots, cut in bite-size pieces

1 cup (250 mL) celery, cut in bite-size pieces

¾ cup (175 mL) brown rice

¾ cup (175 mL) barley (omit if you want to make this gluten-free)

Sea salt, pepper and any herbs you like (such as oregano or parsley)

1 to 2 cups (250 to 500 mL) diced cooked chicken

In a large pot, heat chicken stock. Add tomatoes with their juice. Add a little water if you want to change the consistency or the taste of the broth.

In a separate pot, melt coconut oil over medium-high heat. Sauté onion and garlic for a few minutes. Add carrots and celery; sauté for 4 more minutes. Add sautéed vegetables, brown rice and barley to the stock. Season to taste with salt, pepper and herbs. Simmer over medium to low heat for a few hours, until the veggies, brown rice and barley are fully cooked. Stir in cooked chicken; simmer until chicken is heated through.

This soup can be put into jars and frozen, but it's so good you will probably want to eat it all in one week. Make sure you leave ½ to 1 inch (1 to 2.5 cm) between the top of the soup and the rim of the jar to allow room for the liquid to expand when it freezes.

Joyous Tip

There are times when we crave chicken soup, but it isn't just for its warmth and comfort; there is some good science behind that craving. (I love when science proves that something we innately know is good for us really is!) A 2000 study at the University of Nebraska found that chicken soup may contain anti-inflammatory properties, which help soothe a cold. The experts concluded that something in chicken soup inhibited the movement of neutrophils, white blood cells that are released in great numbers during viral infections (such as a cold) and that lead to mucus, coughing and a stuffy nose. The researchers wrote that "chicken soup may contain a number of substances with beneficial medicinal activity."

Carrot Ginger Soup with Lemon Tahini Drizzle

This easy carrot soup is made from kitchen staples, so it's a great choice when you don't have much in the kitchen but want to eat something homemade and healthy.

Serves 4 to 6

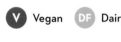 **Vegan**   **DF** **Dairy-free**   **GF** **Gluten-free**

2 tbsp (30 mL) coconut oil

1-inch (2.5 cm) piece fresh ginger, peeled and chopped

4 cloves garlic, chopped

1 lb (450 g) carrots, peeled and chopped

4 cups (1 L) vegetable broth

Salt and pepper

Drizzle

¼ cup (60 mL) tahini

Juice of ½ lemon

1 clove garlic, minced

2 tbsp (30 mL) water

Melt coconut oil in a large saucepan over medium-high heat. Add ginger and garlic; sauté for 1 minute. Add carrots and continue to sauté for 4 to 5 minutes or until slightly softened. Add vegetable broth. Increase heat to bring the soup to a boil. Once it is boiling, lower the heat and simmer until the vegetables are tender, 20 to 25 minutes.

Purée the soup with an immersion blender or in a regular blender. Season with salt and pepper.

For the drizzle, combine all ingredients in a small bowl and whisk to blend. Season with salt and pepper.

Reheat soup if needed. Pour soup into bowls and drizzle with tahini dressing.

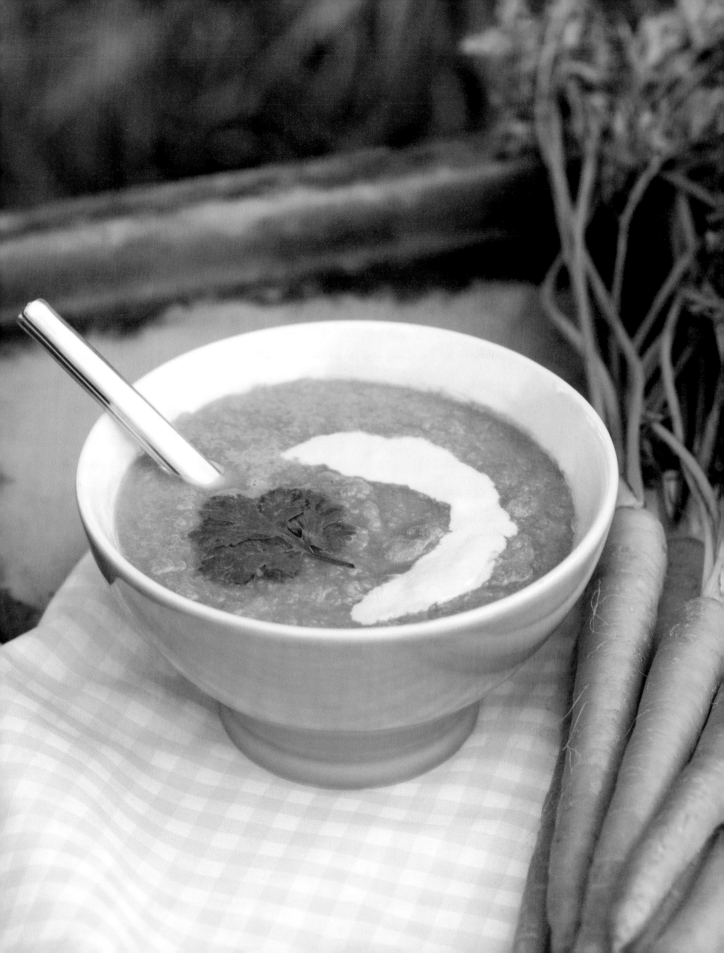

Chilled Cucumber Avocado Soup

While traveling in Mexico I came across a tiny and very rustic roadside restaurant where an elderly lady cooked in the open kitchen. I sat down, and she told me in broken English that she knew exactly what I needed—this soup! It's perfect for a hot summer day. As soon as I was back in Canada I recreated it because it was so refreshingly delicious and easy.

Serves 3 or 4

(V) **Vegetarian**   (GF) **Gluten-free**

2 ripe avocados, peeled and cut in large chunks

1 small cucumber, cut in large chunks, reserving some thin slices for garnish

1 clove garlic

1 cup (250 mL) plain yogurt (or coconut milk yogurt for a dairy-free option)

¼ cup (60 mL) fresh dill

¼ cup (60 mL) cilantro

Juice of 2 limes

Place all ingredients in a food processor and process until smooth and creamy. If you prefer a creamier texture, add more yogurt. Garnish with slices of cucumber and chill for 30 minutes before serving.

Chicken or Turkey Stock

Making your own stock may seem like an overwhelming task, but it's easier than you might think. Whenever I roast a chicken or turkey, I make stock with the leftover carcass because it provides the most flavorful base for all your soups.

Makes about 7 cups (1.75 L)

(DF) **Dairy-free**   (GF) **Gluten-free**

1 chicken or turkey carcass

3 onions, roughly chopped

3 cloves garlic

2 stalks celery

2 carrots

8 cups (2 L) filtered water or enough to cover the carcass

Place the carcass, onions, garlic, celery and carrots in a large soup pot. Add filtered water to cover the carcass. Bring to a gentle boil, then reduce heat and simmer, without stirring, for 1 to 2 hours, skimming any foam from the surface.

Remove from heat and let cool. Cover and refrigerate overnight to let the flavors mingle.

The next day, you may skim off the solidified fat, although this is where most of the flavor is contained. Strain the stock, discarding the solids. Stock keeps, refrigerated, for 5 days or can be frozen for a few months.

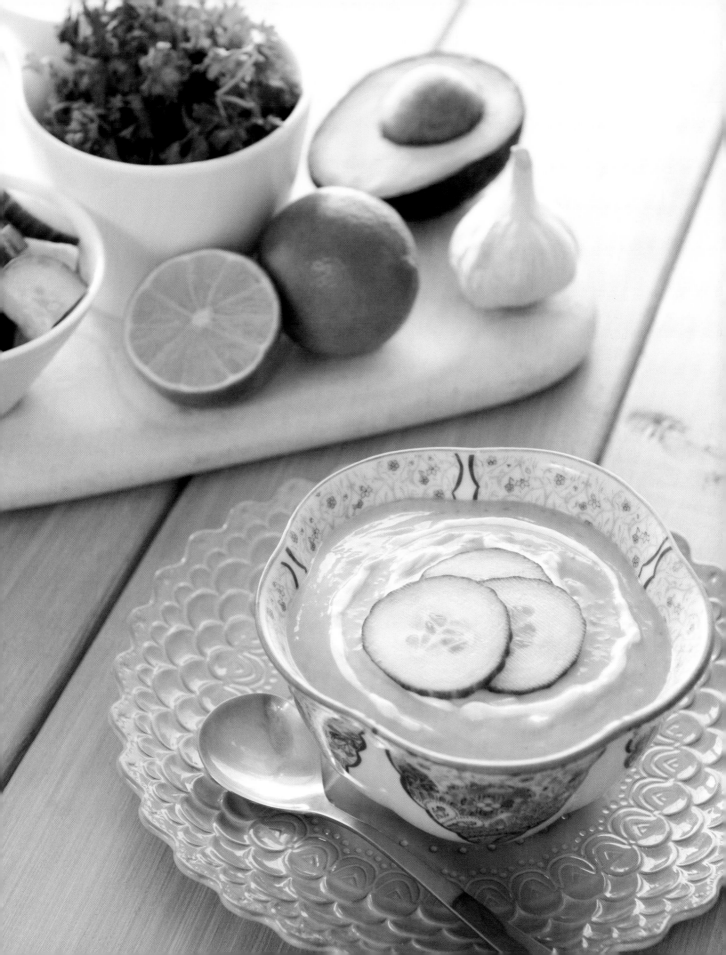

Summer Lovin' Gazpacho

I love picking tomatoes in the summer from my mom's organic garden in Chatsworth, Ontario. When tomatoes are in season, this fresh and vibrant soup is as good as one any five-star chef could create in a restaurant, and you can make it in your own joyous kitchen!

Serves 4

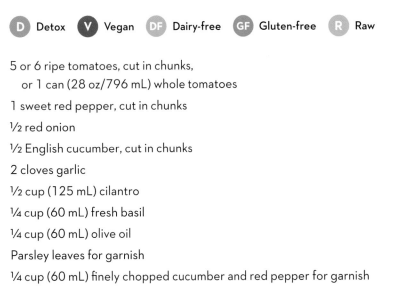 Detox   Vegan   Dairy-free   Gluten-free   Raw

5 or 6 ripe tomatoes, cut in chunks,
    or 1 can (28 oz/796 mL) whole tomatoes

1 sweet red pepper, cut in chunks

½ red onion

½ English cucumber, cut in chunks

2 cloves garlic

½ cup (125 mL) cilantro

¼ cup (60 mL) fresh basil

¼ cup (60 mL) olive oil

Parsley leaves for garnish

¼ cup (60 mL) finely chopped cucumber and red pepper for garnish

Place all the ingredients except the garnishes in a blender or food processor. Process to your desired consistency (I like a few soft chunks). Refrigerate for up to 1 hour. Serve chilled with a garnish of parsley and a touch of finely chopped cucumber and red pepper.

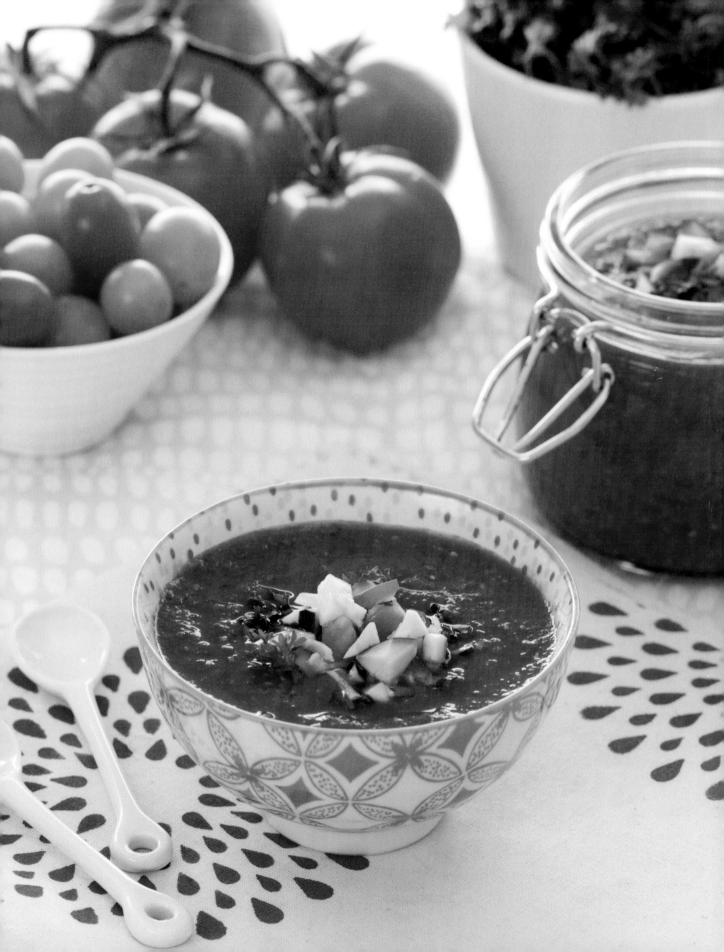

Cardamom Parsnip Pear Soup

The sweetness of pear softens the distinct taste of the parsnips, and the cardamom adds a wonderfully comforting flavor—it's a match made in joyous heaven! The garnish of hemp seeds adds a splash of protein.

Serves 4 to 6

 V Vegan   **DF** Dairy-free   **GF** Gluten-free

2 or 3 medium parsnips, peeled if not organic, cut in chunks

2 Bosc pears, peeled if not organic, cored and cut in chunks

3 to 4 cups (750 mL to 1 L) almond milk or water

1 to 2 tsp (5 to 10 mL) ground cardamom

Lots of freshly cracked black pepper and a pinch of sea salt

¾ cup (175 mL) hemp seeds for garnish

Preheat oven to 350°F (180°C). Place parsnips in a covered baking dish with ½ inch (1 cm) of water. Do the same in a separate dish with the pears. Bake, covered, until parsnips and pears are fork-tender. The pears will take about 35 minutes and the parsnips may take up to an hour.

Transfer pears, parsnips and any liquid from the dishes to a food processor or blender. Add almond milk and cardamom. Process until smooth. (Or transfer to a large saucepan and blend with an immersion blender.) Transfer to a large saucepan and bring to a gentle boil. Remove from heat. Season with pepper and salt. Garnish with hemp seeds.

Quick Method: If you are crunched for time and have a super-high-powered blender like a Vitamix, place all the raw ingredients except salt, pepper and hemp seeds in the blender and blend until smooth. Transfer to a large saucepan and bring to a gentle boil. Reduce heat and simmer for 10 minutes. Season with pepper and salt, and garnish with hemp seeds.

Joyous Tip

Parsnips and potatoes have many of the same health benefits. Actually, parsnips were a major staple in Europe until the late nineteenth century, when they were upstaged by the blander but more versatile potato. They are an excellent source of fiber, vitamin C, folic acid (more than potatoes), manganese and copper. Parsnips are also a good source of B vitamins (thiamine, niacin, riboflavin), magnesium and potassium.

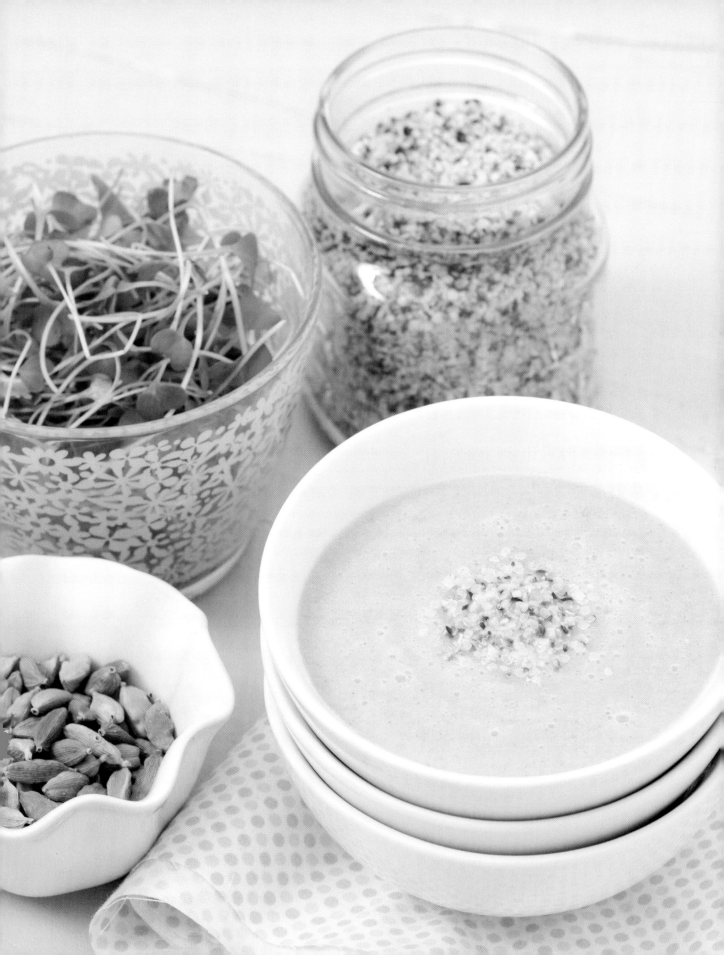

Mama Bea's Curry Lentil Soup

A few years ago, my boyfriend, Walker (now my hubby), texted me a photo of a very old looking wrinkled piece of paper with a handwritten recipe for lentil soup. Walker asked, "Would this be a joy-approved recipe? It's Mama Bea's"—that's Walker's grandma. It was definitely approved—and it's become a favorite!

Serves 4 to 6

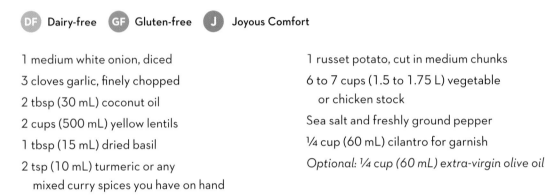 **DF** Dairy-free   **GF** Gluten-free   **J** Joyous Comfort

1 medium white onion, diced

3 cloves garlic, finely chopped

2 tbsp (30 mL) coconut oil

2 cups (500 mL) yellow lentils

1 tbsp (15 mL) dried basil

2 tsp (10 mL) turmeric or any mixed curry spices you have on hand

1 russet potato, cut in medium chunks

6 to 7 cups (1.5 to 1.75 L) vegetable or chicken stock

Sea salt and freshly ground pepper

¼ cup (60 mL) cilantro for garnish

Optional: ¼ cup (60 mL) extra-virgin olive oil

In a large soup pot over medium heat, cook onion and garlic in coconut oil, stirring frequently, until tender. Using a sieve, rinse lentils under running water. Add to vegetables along with basil, turmeric and potato. Pour in 6 cups (1.5 L) of the stock. Bring to a boil, reduce heat and simmer until lentils are tender, 20 to 30 minutes. Add more stock if you prefer a thinner soup.

Season with sea salt and pepper. Serve garnished with cilantro. While you are salivating with anticipation, drizzle with some olive oil for a healthy dose of monounsaturated fat, if you wish.

Joyous Tip

If you want this recipe to be truly gluten-free, make sure any packaged dried spices you use do not contain any gluten.

Thai Beet Soup

The earthy and natural sweetness of beets combine joyously with Thai flavors. Beets are truly a superfood with their mixture of unusual antioxidants.

Serves 4 to 6

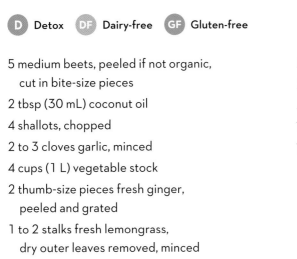 **D** Detox **DF** Dairy-free **GF** Gluten-free

5 medium beets, peeled if not organic,
   cut in bite-size pieces

2 tbsp (30 mL) coconut oil

4 shallots, chopped

2 to 3 cloves garlic, minced

4 cups (1 L) vegetable stock

2 thumb-size pieces fresh ginger,
   peeled and grated

1 to 2 stalks fresh lemongrass,
   dry outer leaves removed, minced

2 cups (500 mL) coconut milk

2 tbsp (30 mL) Thai fish sauce

Juice of 2 limes

½ tsp (2 mL) salt

¼ cup (60 mL) cilantro

Preheat oven to 350°F (180°C). Place beets in a baking dish and add just enough water to cover the bottom of the dish. Cover and bake until beets are fork-tender, about 45 minutes.

Meanwhile, in a large pot over medium heat, melt coconut oil. Cook shallots and garlic for a few minutes, stirring frequently. Add stock, ginger and lemongrass. Once the beets are cooked, add them to the pot. Add coconut milk, fish sauce, lime juice and salt. Simmer until heated through. Garnish each bowl of soup with cilantro.

Option: You may prefer a puréed soup. Once all the ingredients are in the pot, blend until smooth with an immersion blender.

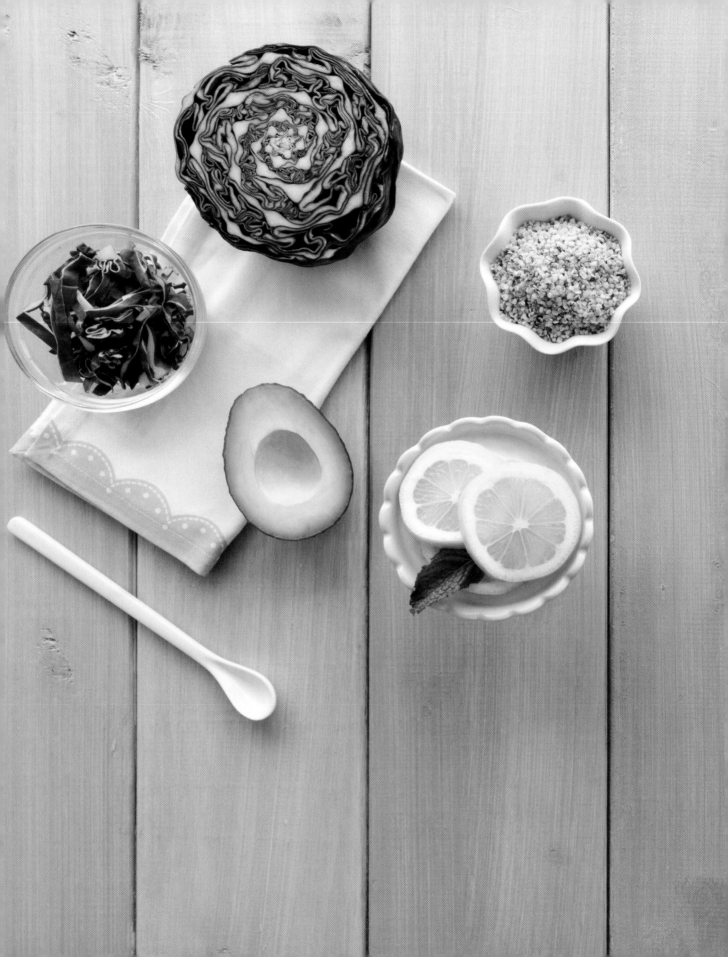

SALADS AND SNACKS

Chickpea Detox Salad   193

Dijon Honey Dressing   193

Keep It Simple Detox Dressing   193

Grilled Veggie Quinoa Salad   194

Creamy Herb Potato Salad   197

Mango Cashew Millet Salad with Lime Ginger Vinaigrette   198

Apple Beet Carrot Slaw with Honey Dressing   200

Kale Orange Pecan Salad   202

Farmers' Market Bruschetta   205

Lemon Pumpkin Seed Sea Salt Kale Chips   206

Curry-Spiced Kale Chips   206

Cheesy Kale Chips   208

Sun-Dried Tomato Hummus   209

Hemp Seed Guacamole   210

Turmeric Sea Salt Popcorn   212

Superfood Trail Mix   215

Almond Power Muffins   217

Chewy Almond Butter Cookies   219

Hemp Seed Maple Cinnamon Butter   220

Beet Goat Cheese Dip   222

Almond Flour Rosemary Crackers   222

Chickpea Detox Salad

This crunchy salad is a summertime favorite of mine. It's so quick and easy to make and keeps in the fridge for at least a week. The fiber and phytonutrients make this an ideal detox meal. Chickpeas are a natural appetite suppressant too!

Serves 2

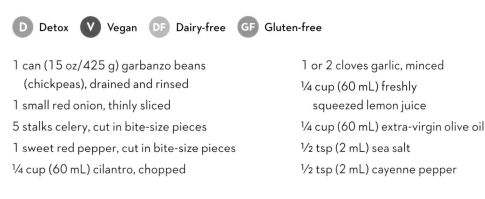 Detox Vegan Dairy-free Gluten-free

1 can (15 oz/425 g) garbanzo beans
   (chickpeas), drained and rinsed

1 small red onion, thinly sliced

5 stalks celery, cut in bite-size pieces

1 sweet red pepper, cut in bite-size pieces

¼ cup (60 mL) cilantro, chopped

1 or 2 cloves garlic, minced

¼ cup (60 mL) freshly
   squeezed lemon juice

¼ cup (60 mL) extra-virgin olive oil

½ tsp (2 mL) sea salt

½ tsp (2 mL) cayenne pepper

Combine all ingredients in a large bowl; toss well. Let sit for an hour so the flavors can mingle.

Salad Dressing

Dijon Honey Dressing

Detox Vegetarian

Dairy-free Gluten-free

¼ cup (60 mL) filtered water

3 tbsp (60 mL) extra-virgin olive oil

2 tbsp (30 mL) Dijon mustard

1 to 2 tbsp (15 to 30 mL) raw honey

Juice of ½ lemon

Combine all ingredients in a small bowl and whisk until emulsified (or shake in a jar).

Keep It Simple Detox Dressing

Detox Vegan

Dairy-free Gluten-free

½ cup (125 mL) hemp oil or extra-virgin olive oil

¼ cup (60 mL) cilantro, chopped

½ clove garlic, minced

Juice of 2 lemons

Pinch of sea salt

Combine all ingredients in a small bowl and whisk until emulsified (or shake in a jar).

Double or triple ingredients for more than two people.

Grilled Veggie Quinoa Salad

This recipe is perfect for BBQ season because it's fresh and full of seasonal ingredients. So instead of buying coleslaw or a bean salad full of salt and processed vegetable oil, take a few minutes and make this heart-healthy quinoa salad. Quinoa is an excellent vegetarian source of protein.

Serves 4

D Detox **V** Vegetarian **GF** Gluten-free

1 cup (250 mL) quinoa (any color)

3 sweet peppers (any color), coarsely chopped

1 yellow zucchini, coarsely chopped

1 red onion, cut in wedges

1 tbsp (15 mL) extra-virgin olive oil

4 cups (1 L) arugula or chopped kale

2 tbsp (30 mL) crumbled goat cheese

Optional: ¼ cup (60 mL) chopped parsley

Dressing

2 tbsp (30 mL) freshly squeezed lemon juice

1 tbsp (15 mL) cider vinegar

1 tbsp (15 mL) grainy Dijon mustard

½ cup (125 mL) extra-virgin olive oil

1 clove garlic, minced

½ tsp (2 mL) sea salt

Cook the quinoa according to the recipe on page 137; transfer to a large bowl. Preheat grill to medium-high.

Lightly toss peppers, zucchini and onion with oil. Grill, turning occasionally, until tender, 6 to 8 minutes. Add to quinoa and toss well.

Combine dressing ingredients in a bowl (or jar), whisking (or shaking) until emulsified. You can double or triple the dressing recipe if you prefer more flavor. Toss with salad. Let cool slightly. Toss with arugula, then sprinkle with goat cheese. Garnish with parsley if using.

· ·

Joyous Tip

If there are any leftovers, this salad is just as tasty the next day. Keep refrigerated.

· ·

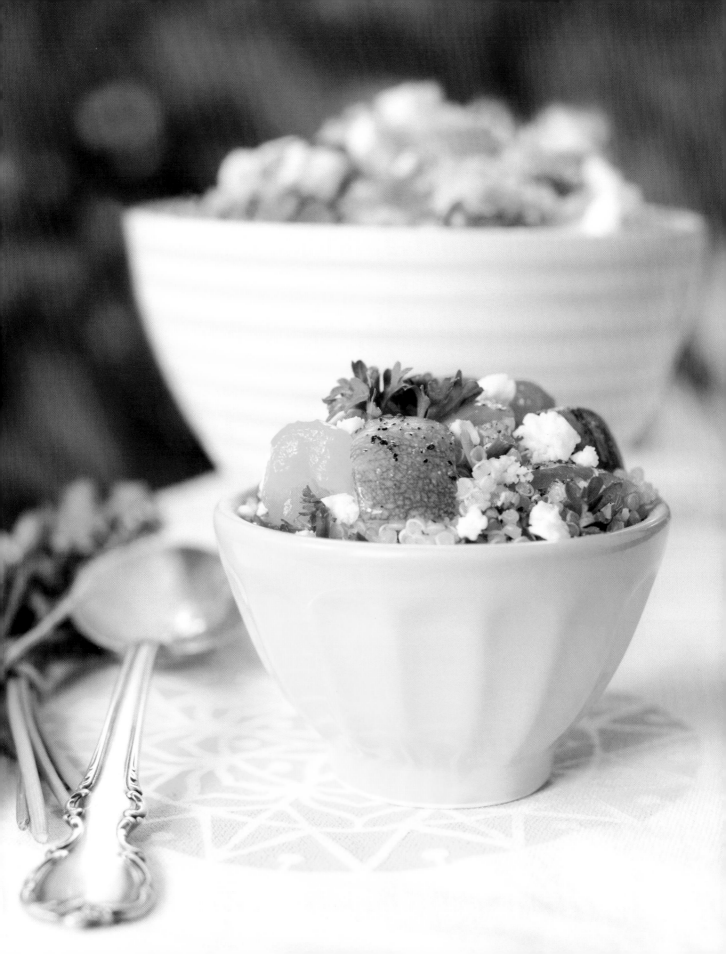

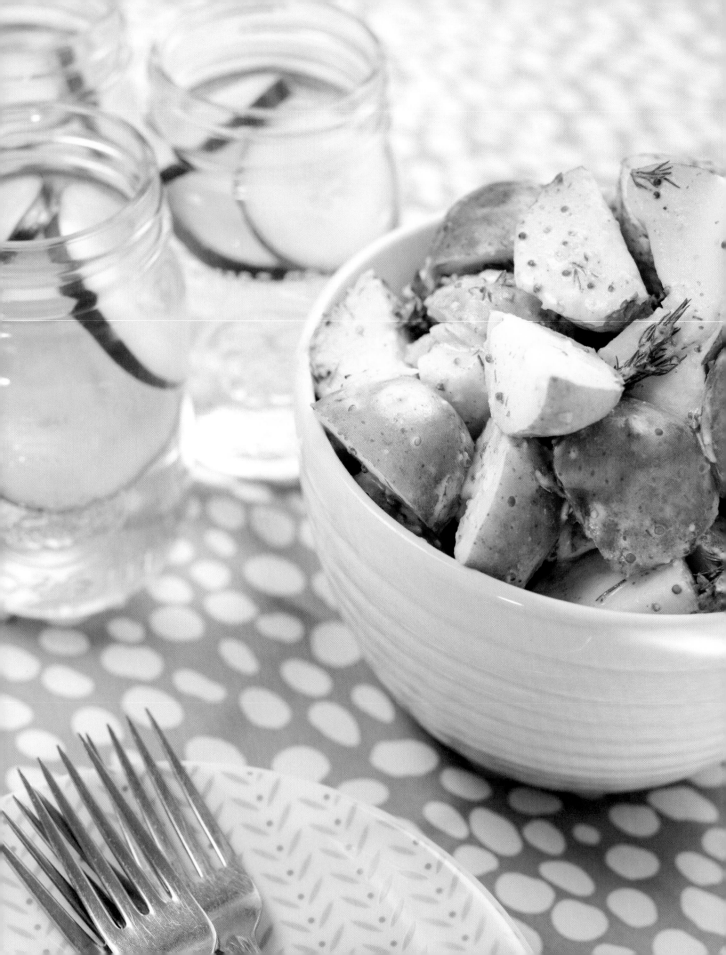

Creamy Herb Potato Salad

If you love potato salad as much as I do but had to give it up because you have trouble digesting dairy or don't like a mayonnaise-drenched salad, this recipe will come as a healthy surprise. It's proof positive that healthy can and should be delicious! I love surprising family and friends with this recipe. No one ever believes me that it's healthy!

Serves 4

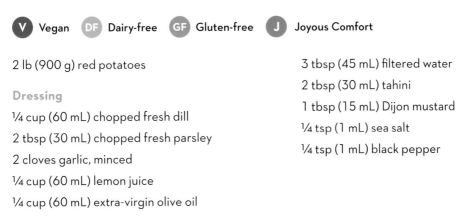

V Vegan   **DF** Dairy-free   **GF** Gluten-free   **J** Joyous Comfort

2 lb (900 g) red potatoes

Dressing

¼ cup (60 mL) chopped fresh dill

2 tbsp (30 mL) chopped fresh parsley

2 cloves garlic, minced

¼ cup (60 mL) lemon juice

¼ cup (60 mL) extra-virgin olive oil

3 tbsp (45 mL) filtered water

2 tbsp (30 mL) tahini

1 tbsp (15 mL) Dijon mustard

¼ tsp (1 mL) sea salt

¼ tsp (1 mL) black pepper

If you have organic potatoes, you do not need to peel them. Wash and cut potatoes into small chunks. Bring a large pot of water to a gentle boil. Add potatoes and boil just until tender, 15 to 20 minutes. Be careful not to overcook. Drain and run under cold water; drain again. Let cool completely.

In a large bowl, whisk together dressing ingredients until well combined. Toss potatoes with dressing. Refrigerate for a few hours and serve chilled.

Joyous Tip

The skin of the potato is nutrient-dense and contains most of the phytonutrients, which is why I suggest you do not peel them.

On a hot summer's day enjoy this salad with Curry Chicken Burgers (page 227) for a nutritious and complete meal.

Mango Cashew Millet Salad with Lime Ginger Vinaigrette

I was inspired by my favorite take-out salad from Sukho Thai in Toronto to create this tangy and full-of-texture salad. The millet makes it a meal unto itself, or you could enjoy it as a starter to the Raw Sunshine Wraps (page 236).

Serves 4

D Detox **V** Vegetarian **DF** Dairy-free **GF** Gluten-free

1½ cups (375 mL) millet

3 cups (750 mL) filtered water

2 mangoes, peeled and cut in small cubes

1 cup (250 mL) raw cashews, coarsely chopped

½ cup (125 mL) finely chopped fresh mint

½ cup (125 mL) finely chopped cilantro

Sea salt and pepper

Parsley for garnish

Dressing

Juice of 2 limes

3 tbsp (45 mL) extra-virgin olive oil

2 tbsp (30 mL) rice vinegar

2 tbsp (30 mL) honey

1 tbsp (15 mL) grated fresh ginger

¼ tsp (1 mL) salt

In a large saucepan, combine millet and filtered water. Bring to a boil, reduce heat to low and simmer, covered and stirring occasionally, for 20 to 25 minutes, until all the water has been absorbed and the millet is fluffy. Remove from heat.

Prepare vinaigrette by whisking together all ingredients in a small bowl.

In a large bowl, combine millet, mangoes, cashews and fresh herbs. Season with salt and pepper. Garnish with parsley. Drizzle with the dressing and toss well. Refrigerate for at least 1 hour. Serve chilled.

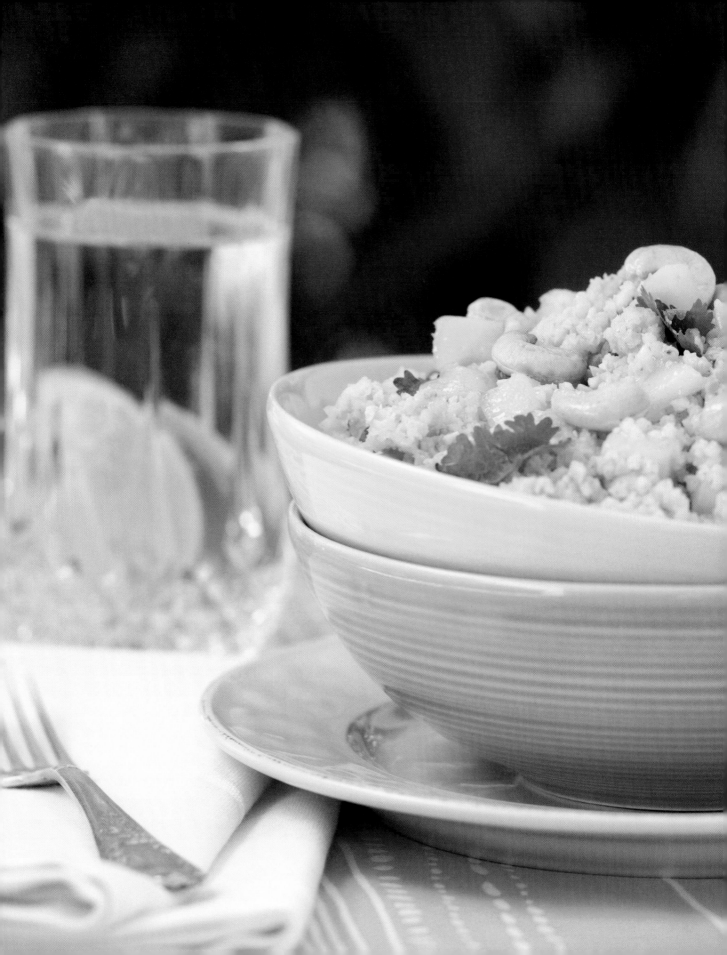

Apple Beet Carrot Slaw with Honey Dressing

Fresh, vibrant and full of flavor, this completely raw slaw will not only love your liver—it's bursting with fiber and detoxifying nutrients—but it will energize you too. I enjoy this slaw with some grilled fish or topped with hemp seeds as a vegetarian dish.

Serves 4

D Detox   **V** Vegetarian   **DF** Dairy-free   **GF** Gluten-free

2 apples (unpeeled if organic), chopped in bite-size pieces

4 carrots, grated

3 beets, trimmed and grated

2 tbsp (30 mL) honey

2 tbsp (30 mL) cider vinegar

2 tbsp (30 mL) extra-virgin olive oil

½ tsp (2 mL) sea salt

Optional: ½ cup (125 mL) chopped fresh parsley or cilantro for garnish

In a large bowl, stir together apples, carrots and beets. In a small bowl, whisk together honey, vinegar, oil and sea salt until emulsified. Just before serving, toss dressing with the slaw. Garnish with parsley if using.

Joyous Tip

If you don't want the beets to turn the apples red, add the beets just before serving.

You don't have to peel any of your produce if you buy all organic and wash it well.

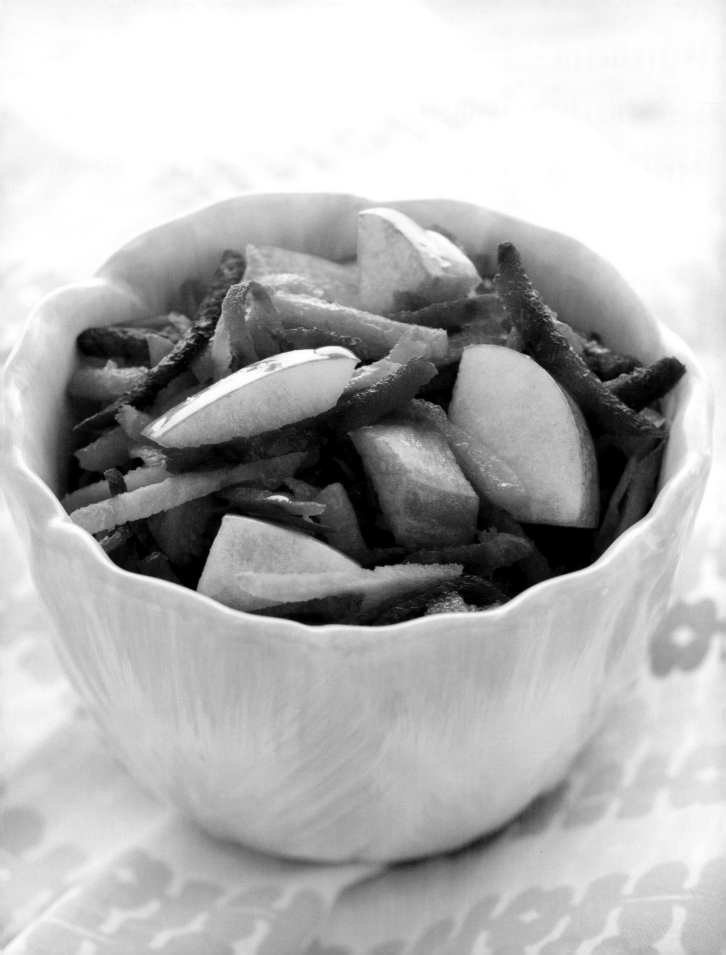

Kale Orange Pecan Salad

This amazing salad is bursting with vitamin C, carotenoids and fiber, making it immune boosting. The oranges give it a wonderful sweet flavor, and the pecans add a nice crunchy bite.

Serves 4

D Detox   **DF** Dairy-free   **GF** Gluten-free

1 bunch kale, washed and patted dry
2 oranges, peeled and sliced crosswise
½ cup (125 mL) pecans

Dressing
½ cup (125 mL) brown rice vinegar
⅓ cup (75 mL) sesame oil
¼ cup (60 mL) orange-flavored omega-3 fish oil
½ cup (125 mL) fresh mint leaves
2 tbsp (30 mL) grated orange zest
Juice of 1 orange

Tear kale away from the stems and tear into bite-size pieces. Place in a large bowl.

Combine all the dressing ingredients in a food processor; process until the mint is completely chopped, about 30 seconds. Pour dressing over the kale and toss well. Arrange orange slices on top and sprinkle with pecans.

· ·

Joyous Tip

Flavored fish oil does not have a fishy taste. In fact, there are brands of fish oil that taste like orange (per this recipe, Genuine Health) or even lemon. If you don't have this or you are vegan, use hemp or flaxseed oil.

· ·

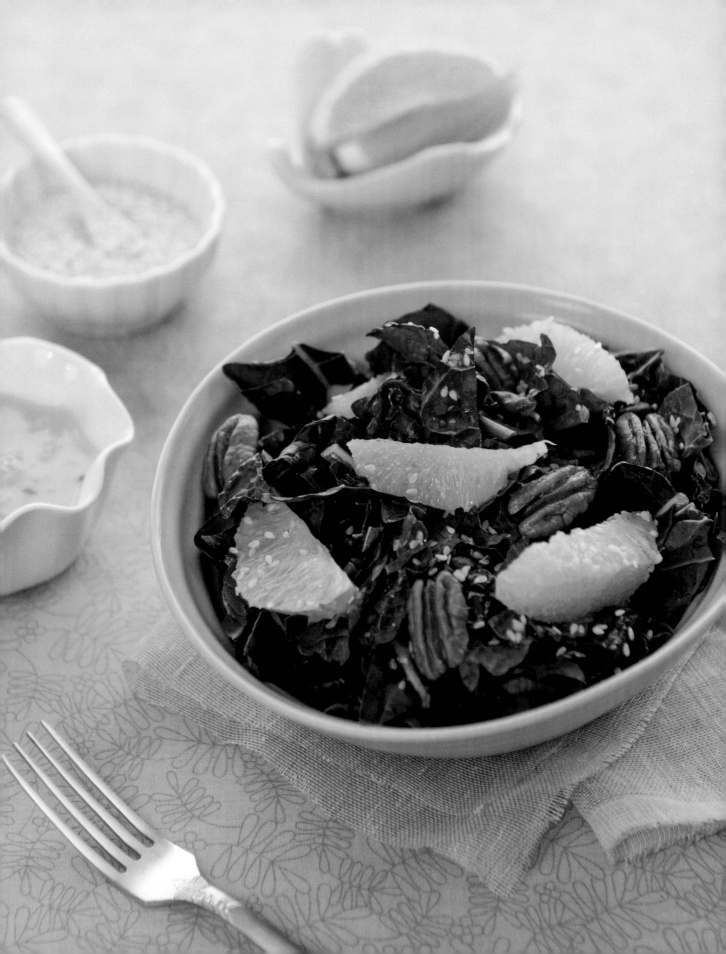

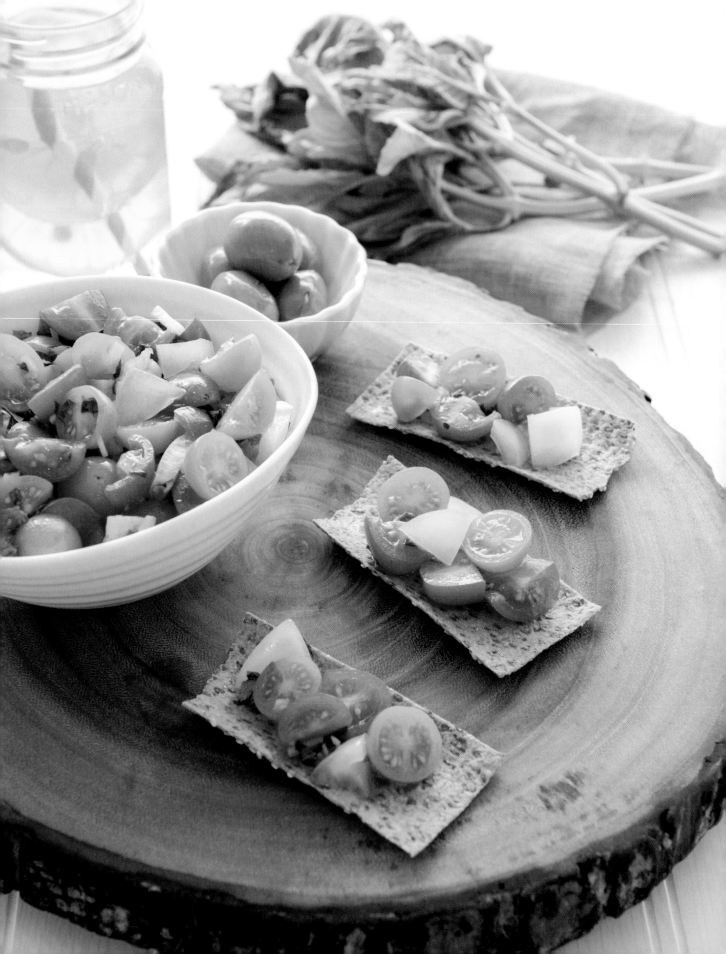

Farmers' Market Bruschetta

Serve this at your party along with Hemp Seed Guacamole (page 210) and some Sangria Kombucha (page 166) and your guests will be wanting to know when your next get-together is going to be!

Serves 2 to 4

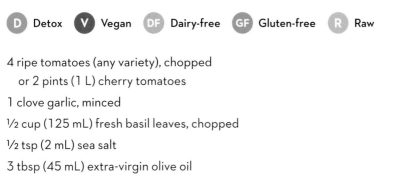

D Detox   **V** Vegan   **DF** Dairy-free   **GF** Gluten-free   **R** Raw

4 ripe tomatoes (any variety), chopped
   or 2 pints (1 L) cherry tomatoes
1 clove garlic, minced
½ cup (125 mL) fresh basil leaves, chopped
½ tsp (2 mL) sea salt
3 tbsp (45 mL) extra-virgin olive oil

Combine all ingredients in a bowl; toss well. Let marinate for at least 10 minutes. Serve on crackers—perhaps the Almond Flour Rosemary Crackers on page 222—with some fresh olives.

Kale Chips
Three Delicious Ways

I'm convinced I can turn most anyone into a kale-chip-lover. I have evidence. Although he might not want to admit it, my girlfriend's ten-year-old boy devours them every time he starts munching on some! If you are a newbie to kale chips, they are dehydrated bite-size pieces of kale with various concoctions of deliciousness. Basically, they will take on the taste of the seasoning. My three favorite variations will satisfy even the most finicky eater. Each recipe serves 2 to 4 as a snack. Kale chips keep in an airtight container for 1 week.

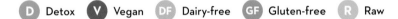

D Detox   **V** Vegan   **DF** Dairy-free   **GF** Gluten-free   **R** Raw

Lemon Pumpkin Seed Sea Salt Kale Chips

1 bunch kale, washed and patted dry

1 tbsp (15 mL) extra-virgin olive oil

Juice of ½ lemon

1 tsp (5 mL) sea salt

2 tbsp (30 mL) unsalted raw pumpkin seeds

Preheat oven to its lowest setting.

Tear kale away from the tough stems and tear into large bite-size pieces. Place in a large bowl. Drizzle with oil and lemon juice; massage into the kale pieces with your hands for a minute or two. Spread kale evenly in a single layer, slightly overlapping if necessary, on a parchment-lined baking sheet. Sprinkle with sea salt and pumpkin seeds.

Bake for 2 to 4 hours or until kale chips are crispy.

Curry-Spiced Kale Chips

1 bunch kale, washed and patted dry

1 tbsp (15 mL) extra-virgin olive oil

1 tsp (5 mL) sea salt

2 tsp (10 mL) your favorite curry powder (or 1 tsp/5 mL turmeric, ½ tsp/2 mL ground cumin and ½ tsp/2 mL garlic powder)

Optional: 1 tsp (5 mL) hot chili flakes

Preheat oven to its lowest setting.

Tear kale away from the tough stems and tear into large bite-size pieces. Place in a large bowl. Drizzle with oil and massage into the kale pieces with your hands for a minute or two. Spread kale evenly in a single layer, slightly overlapping if necessary, on a parchment-lined baking sheet. Sprinkle with sea salt, curry powder and chili flakes, if using.

Bake for 2 to 4 hours or until kale chips are crispy.

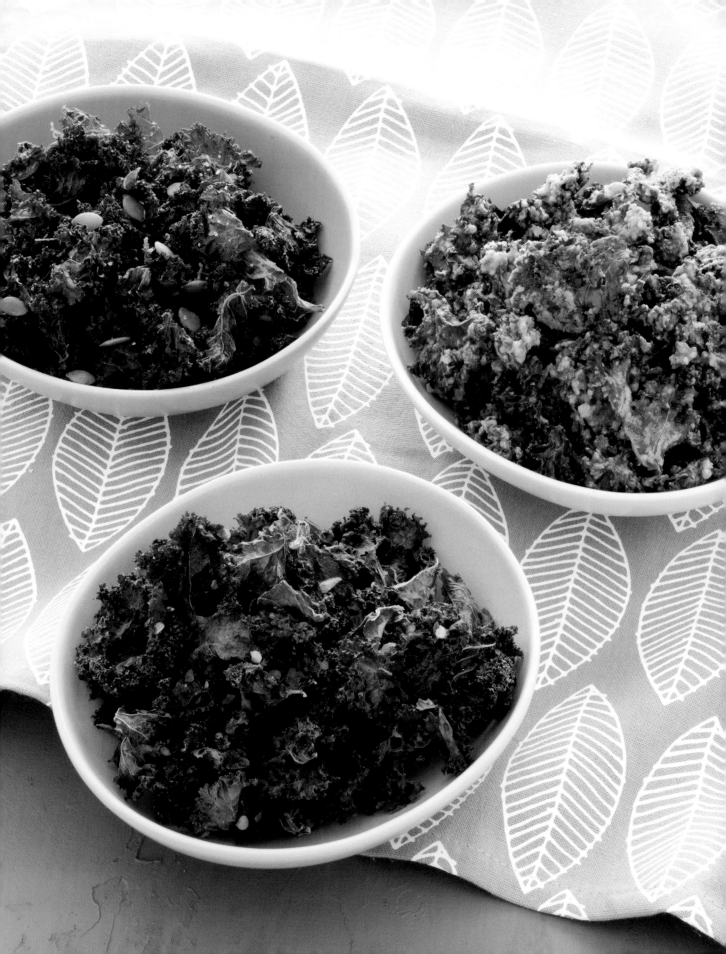

Cheesy Kale Chips

¾ cup (175 mL) raw cashews

1 bunch kale, washed and patted dry

½ sweet red pepper, cut in large pieces

1 clove garlic

⅓ cup (75 mL) nutritional yeast*

2 tbsp (30 mL) extra-virgin olive oil

1 tbsp (15 mL) tamari sauce

Juice of ½ lemon

Nutritional yeast is not the same as yeast used in making bread. Nutritional yeast is a deactivated yeast that gives this recipe a "cheesy" flavor.

In a small bowl, soak cashews in water for at least 1 hour. Drain.

Preheat oven to its lowest setting. Meanwhile, tear kale away from the tough stems and tear into large bite-size pieces. Place in a large bowl.

In a food processor, combine cashews, red pepper, garlic, nutritional yeast, oil and tamari. Process into a paste. Add lemon juice and process until smooth.

Add cashew paste to kale and massage it over kale with your hands, making sure kale is evenly coated. Spread kale evenly in a single layer on a parchment-lined baking sheet, making sure they do not touch. Cover and refrigerate remaining kale until first batch has finished baking.

Bake kale, turning once after the first hour, for 2 to 4 hours, until crisp, completely dry and topping doesn't feel chewy or moist.

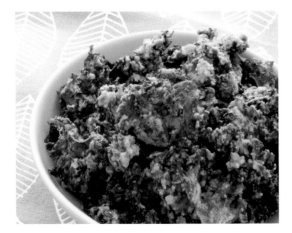

Joyous Tip

Do not overdo the olive oil! While it may seem very little, the kale chips shrink significantly.

Getting impatient waiting? You can turn up the temp to 300°F (150°C), but the chips will finish cooking in 5 to 8 minutes max (depending on how long you've already baked them). Also, cooking at a higher temperature will destroy some of the enzymes and vitamins.

Sun-Dried Tomato Hummus

A perfect addition to your next party along with Hemp Seed Guacamole (page 210) and Farmers' Market Bruschetta (page 205). Your guests will be impressed with your healthy and delicious spread.

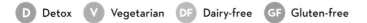

D Detox   **V** Vegetarian   **DF** Dairy-free   **GF** Gluten-free

1 can (15 oz/425 g) garbanzo beans (chickpeas)

5 sun-dried tomatoes*

2 cloves garlic

2 tbsp (30 mL) tahini

¼ cup (60 mL) filtered water

Combine all ingredients in a food processor and process until smooth. Serve with Almond Flour Rosemary Crackers (page 222) or brown rice crackers.

*Look for sulfite-free sun-dried tomatoes

Hemp Seed Guacamole

Always a crowd-pleaser, this guac is a hit at any party. It will probably disappear quite quickly, so you might want to be prepared with an extra batch!

Makes 1½ cups (375 mL)

D Detox **V** Vegan **DF** Dairy-free **GF** Gluten-free

2 ripe avocados
½ medium tomato, finely chopped
½ red onion, finely chopped
1 clove garlic, minced
Juice of 2 limes
½ cup (125 mL) hemp seeds
½ tsp (2 mL) hot sauce (or more if you like it hot)

Spoon avocado flesh from skins and transfer to a bowl. Mash avocado with a fork. Add tomato, red onion, garlic and lime juice. Stir well. Give it a little taste test—add a touch more lime, if needed. Stir in hemp seeds and hot sauce. Serve immediately with blue corn chips or whole wheat pita bread.

· ·

Joyous Tip

Avocados are an amazing source of healthy monounsaturated fats. The hemp seeds are a good source of protein. Protein and fat together make this a very balanced snack.

· ·

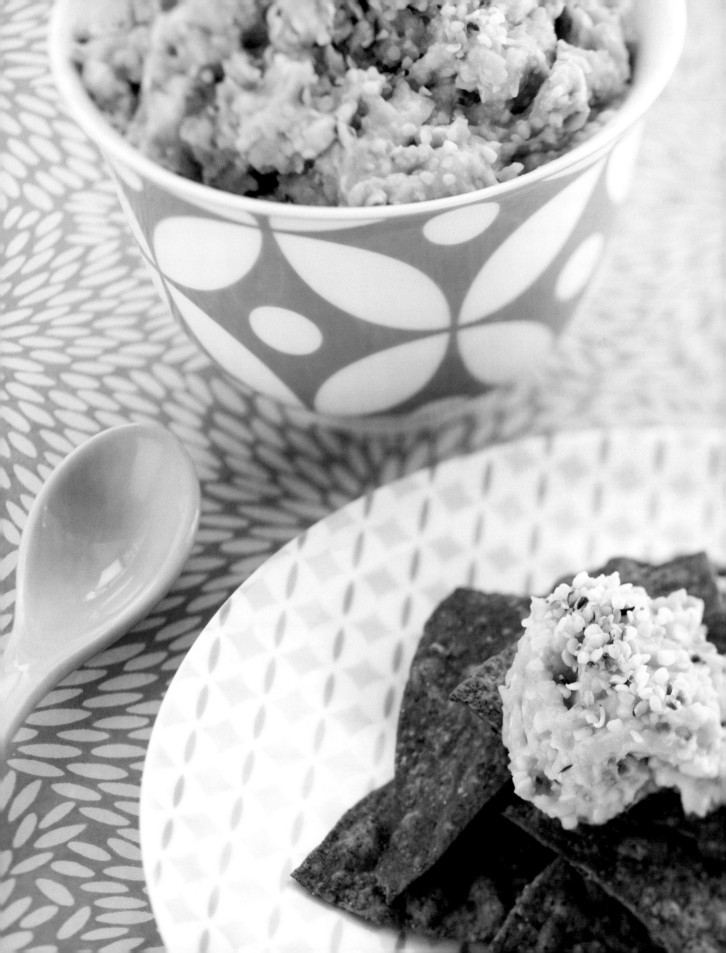

Turmeric Sea Salt Popcorn

What is better than snuggling up with your family on a cold winter's night with a big bowl of popcorn and your favorite movie? I promise you will love this homemade popcorn way more than the microwave version—you will definitely taste the difference!

Makes 4 to 5 cups (1 to 1.25 L)

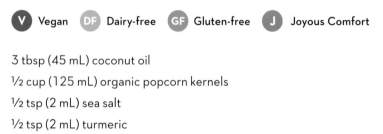 **Vegan** **DF** **Dairy-free** **GF** **Gluten-free** **J** **Joyous Comfort**

3 tbsp (45 mL) coconut oil

½ cup (125 mL) organic popcorn kernels

½ tsp (2 mL) sea salt

½ tsp (2 mL) turmeric

Ground black pepper

In a medium saucepan over medium-high heat, melt coconut oil. Add popcorn kernels. Cover and cook, giving the pot a shake every so often, until you hear the kernels begin to pop. Don't let the pot sit on the hot element for more than 5 or 10 seconds at a time once the kernels begin popping—keep lifting it and giving it a shake. Remove from heat when you hear no more pops. Pour the hot popcorn into a large bowl and sprinkle with sea salt, turmeric and black pepper to taste. Toss well. Serve immediately.

Joyous Tip

Be sure to buy certified organic corn kernels because most corn is genetically modified and highly sprayed with pesticides.

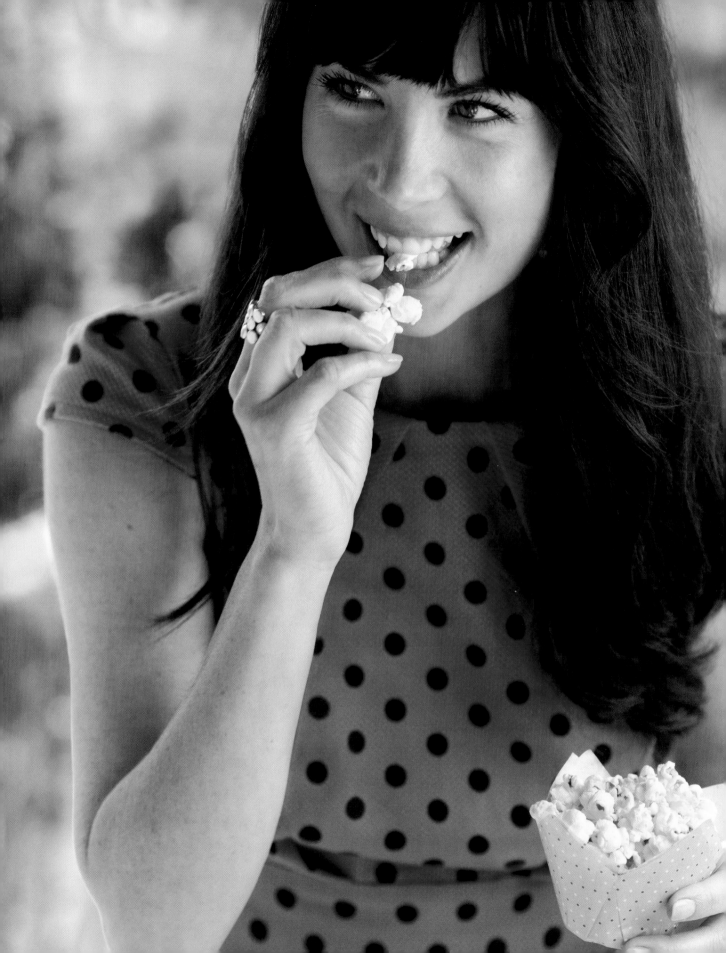

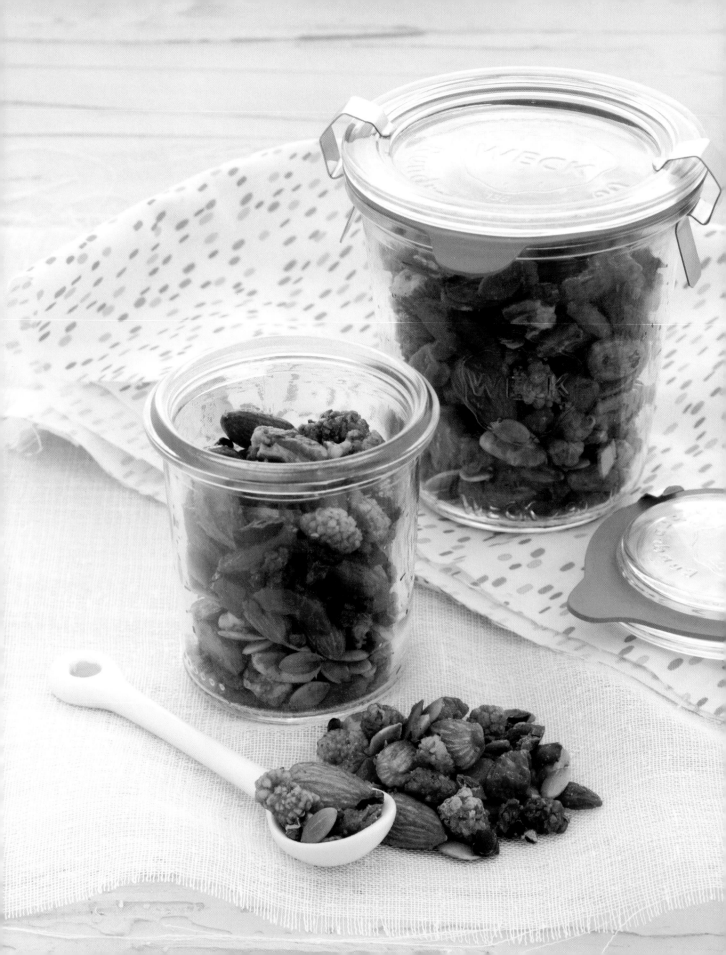

Superfood Trail Mix

My girlfriend Candice helped me create this amazing trail mix for a workshop we were teaching. It was a hit! It's perfect for a hike or a bike ride. Just make sure you have enough to satisfy all the hungry mouths that might be traveling with you!

Makes 4 cups (1 L)

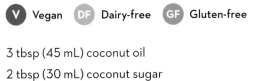 **V** Vegan **DF** Dairy-free **GF** Gluten-free

3 tbsp (45 mL) coconut oil

2 tbsp (30 mL) coconut sugar

1 tsp (5 mL) cinnamon

1 cup (250 mL) pumpkin seeds

¾ cup (175 mL) goji berries

½ cup (125 mL) dried mulberries

½ cup (125 mL) raw almonds

½ cup (125 mL) walnuts

½ cup (125 mL) cacao nibs

In a small pot over low heat, melt coconut oil. Stir in coconut sugar and cinnamon. In a large bowl, stir together the remaining ingredients. Pour oil mixture over top and mix well. Portion out 2 tbsp (30 mL) for an energizing snack!

. . . .

Joyous Tip

This trail mix contains a plethora of goodness! It's all-natural, with none of the additives and preservatives of so many store-bought trail mixes and energy bars.

. . . .

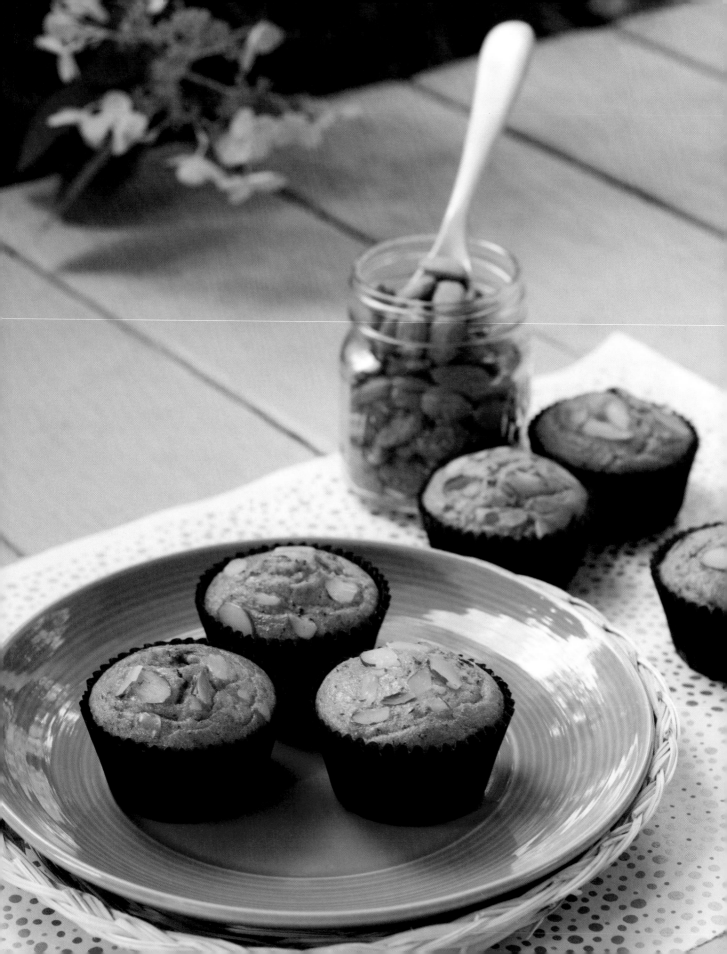

Almond Power Muffins

You'll feel powered up by these satisfying, super-tasty and healthy muffins. The recipe comes from one of my students at the Institute of Holistic Nutrition. He made them for the class and we were energized for hours! They're completely gluten-free and a great source of protein and fiber. Pack them in your bag for a hike or while traveling for a healthy snack.

Makes 12 muffins

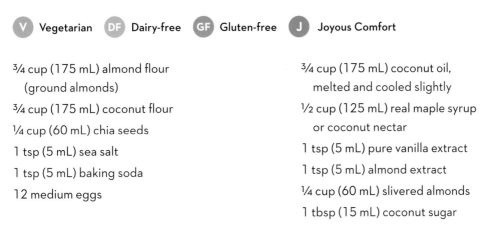 **V** Vegetarian   **DF** Dairy-free   **GF** Gluten-free   **J** Joyous Comfort

¾ cup (175 mL) almond flour
   (ground almonds)

¾ cup (175 mL) coconut flour

¼ cup (60 mL) chia seeds

1 tsp (5 mL) sea salt

1 tsp (5 mL) baking soda

12 medium eggs

¾ cup (175 mL) coconut oil,
   melted and cooled slightly

½ cup (125 mL) real maple syrup
   or coconut nectar

1 tsp (5 mL) pure vanilla extract

1 tsp (5 mL) almond extract

¼ cup (60 mL) slivered almonds

1 tbsp (15 mL) coconut sugar

Preheat oven to 325°F (160°C). Grease a muffin pan or line with paper liners.

In a large bowl, combine almond flour, coconut flour, chia seeds, sea salt and baking soda; mix well. In a separate bowl, whisk the eggs. Add coconut oil, maple syrup, vanilla and almond extract; whisk to blend. Add wet ingredients to dry ingredients and stir just until combined. Do not over-mix.

Spoon batter into muffin cups. Sprinkle with almonds and coconut sugar. Bake for 18 to 20 minutes or until golden brown. Let cool for 10 minutes before removing from pan. Enjoy with some honey.

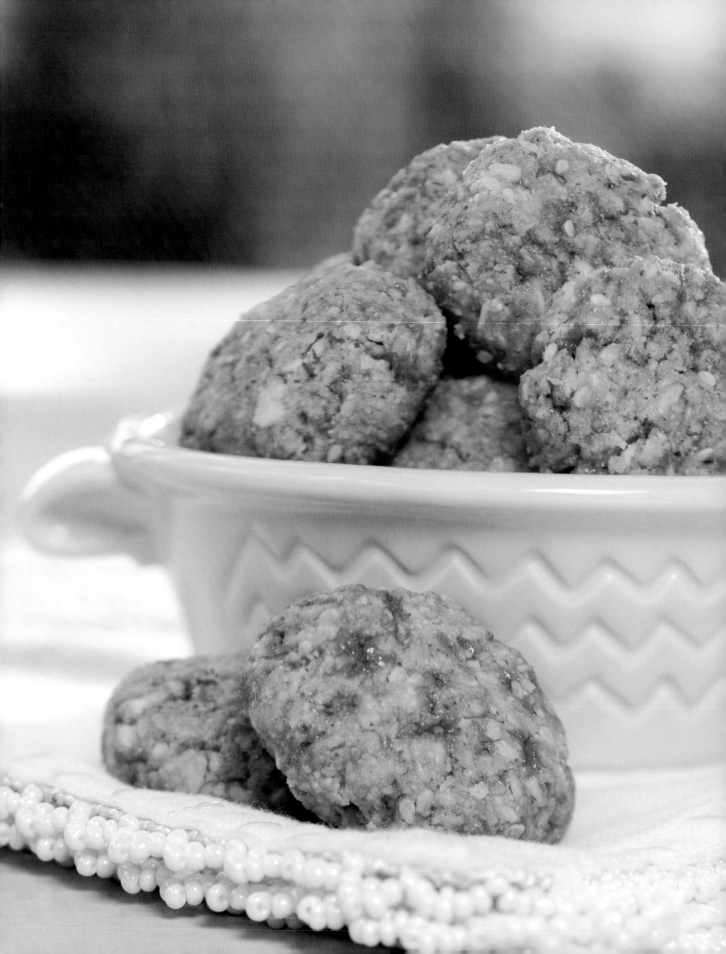

Chewy Almond Butter Cookies

These cookies are a Joyous Health readers' favorite. If you have kids, instead of buying another bag of cookies that have lots of sugar and little nutritional value, make a batch of these and watch your kids devour them. Just make sure you keep some for yourself!

Makes 2 to 3 dozen little gems of deliciousness

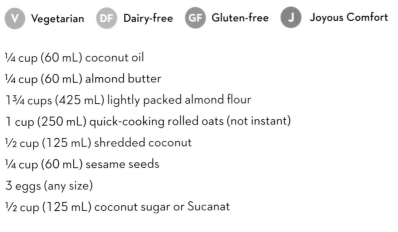 Vegetarian Dairy-free Gluten-free Joyous Comfort

¼ cup (60 mL) coconut oil

¼ cup (60 mL) almond butter

1¾ cups (425 mL) lightly packed almond flour

1 cup (250 mL) quick-cooking rolled oats (not instant)

½ cup (125 mL) shredded coconut

¼ cup (60 mL) sesame seeds

3 eggs (any size)

½ cup (125 mL) coconut sugar or Sucanat

Preheat oven to 350°F (180°C). Grease a cookie sheet.

In a small saucepan over low heat, melt coconut oil and almond butter. Set aside.

In a large bowl, stir together flour, rolled oats, coconut and sesame seeds. In a separate bowl, whisk together eggs and sugar. Add melted oil mixture; mix well. Add wet ingredients to dry ingredients; stir until well mixed.

Form dough into 1-inch (2.5 cm) balls and arrange about 2 inches (5 cm) apart on the cookie sheet. Flatten with a fork. Bake for 10 to 12 minutes or until the edges are golden brown. Transfer cookies to a rack to cool.

Hemp Seed Maple Cinnamon Butter

Healthier than your typical store-bought, sugar-laden peanut butter and a nice alternative to almond butter. Hemp seeds are a true superfood with a smooth, nutty flavor. I enjoy this on toast for breakfast or on crackers as a snack.

Makes 1 cup (250 mL)

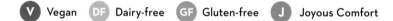 Vegan   DF Dairy-free   GF Gluten-free   J Joyous Comfort

1 cup (250 mL) shelled hemp seeds

2 soft Medjool dates, pitted

3 to 4 tbsp (45 to 60 mL) hemp seed oil

2 to 3 tbsp (30 to 45 mL) dark maple syrup

1 tbsp (15 mL) cinnamon

½ tsp (2 mL) sea salt

Combine all ingredients in a food processor or blender. Process until a paste forms. I like the butter a little chunkier, but you can blend it longer if you prefer it creamier. Serve spread on slices of apple or on toast or crackers. Keeps in the fridge for 2 weeks.

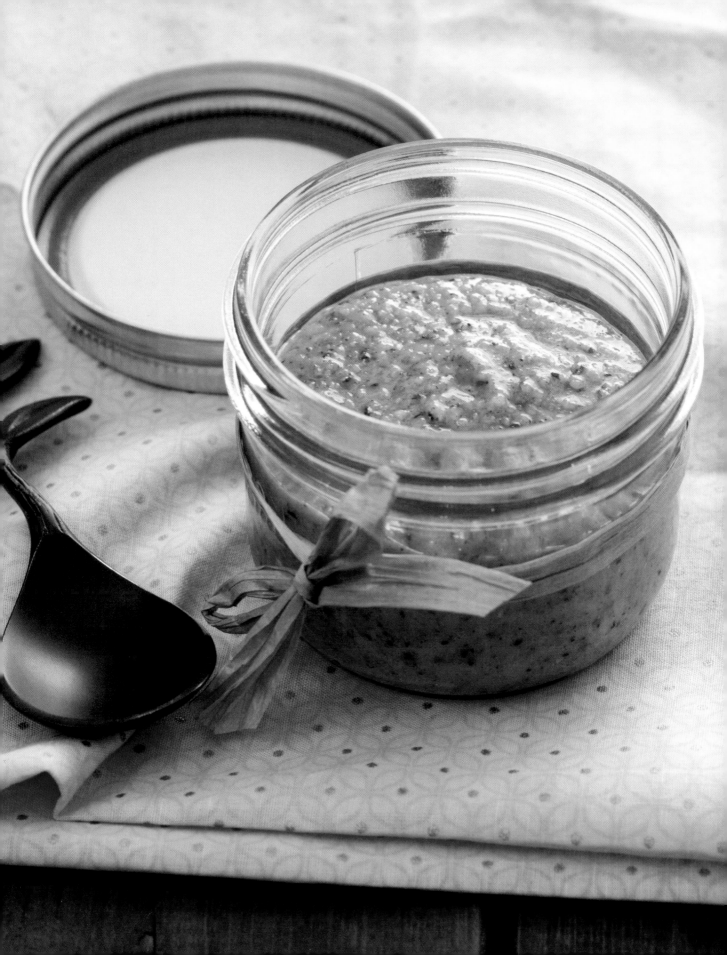

Beet Goat Cheese Dip

The natural sweetness of beets combines beautifully with the richness of goat cheese. When beets are in season, this dip is one of my favorite snacks. Plus, beets are a total superfood!

Makes 2 to 3 cups (500 to 750 mL), depending on size of beets

D Detox   **V** Vegetarian

GF Gluten-free   **J** Joyous Comfort

6 or 7 medium beets, peeled and cut in chunks
1 tbsp (15 mL) grapeseed oil
1 clove garlic
¾ cup (175 mL) soft goat cheese
½ tsp (2 mL) sea salt

Preheat oven to 350°F (180°C).

Place beets in a roasting pan or baking dish with a lid and drizzle with oil. Cover and bake until fork-tender, 35 to 45 minutes, stirring once after 25 minutes. Let cool for 10 to 20 minutes.

In a food processor, combine beets, garlic, goat cheese and sea salt. If your food processor is not large enough, blend in batches. Blend until smooth. Serve with Almond Flour Rosemary Crackers.

Almond Flour Rosemary Crackers

Makes 8 to 10 crackers

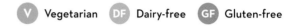

V Vegetarian   **DF** Dairy-free   **GF** Gluten-free

2 cups (500 mL) almond flour (ground almonds)
1½ tsp (7 mL) dried rosemary
2 tsp (10 mL) sea salt
1 medium egg
2 tbsp (30 mL) extra-virgin olive oil

Preheat oven to 350°F (180°C).

In a food processor, combine almond flour, rosemary and salt; pulse to mix. Add egg and oil; pulse just until combined.

Roll out dough as thin as possible between two sheets of parchment paper. Remove the top sheet of paper and slide the other sheet with the dough onto a cookie sheet. (If dough is very soft, put it in the freezer for 10 minutes before cutting.) Use a knife or pizza wheel to cut out 8 to 10 crackers about 1½ inches (4 cm) wide and 3 inches (8 cm) long.

Bake crackers for 10 to 12 minutes or until golden around the edges. Let cool completely on a rack. Serve with Beet Goat Cheese Dip.

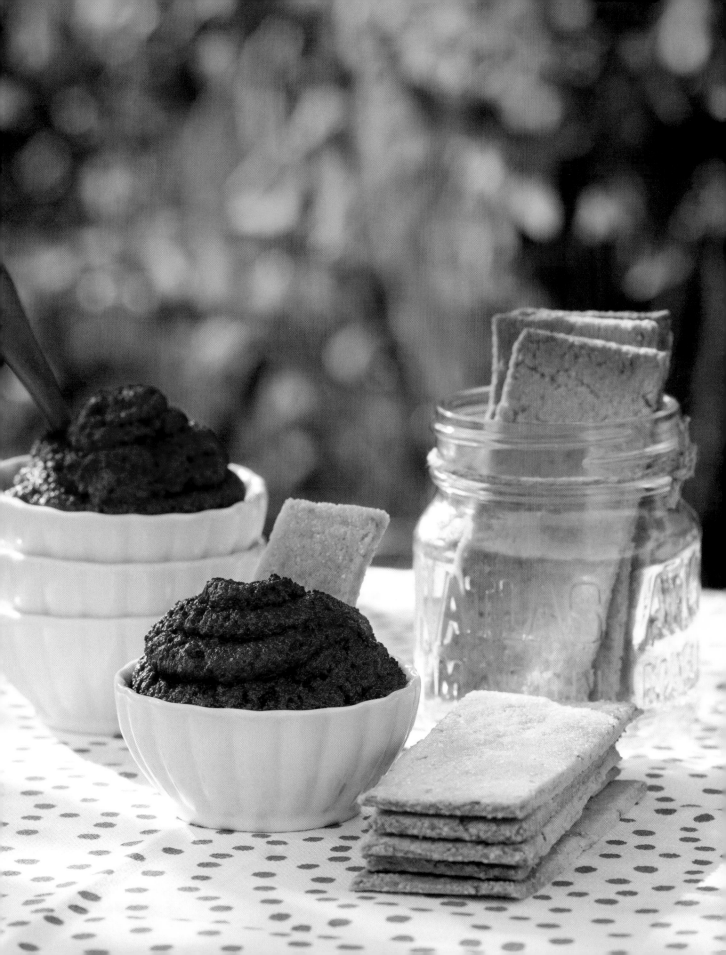

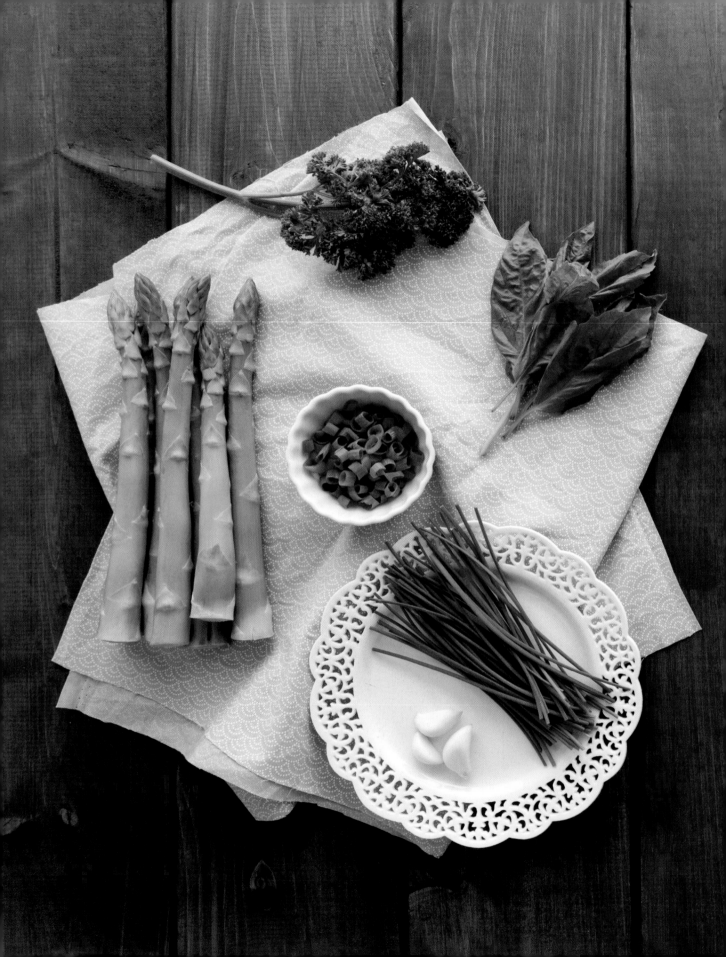

MAINS
AND SIDES

Curry Chicken Burgers with Mango Salsa or Tzatziki   227

Baked Lemon Pepper Salmon with "Cream" Sauce   228

Tamari Broccoli with Sunflower Seeds   230

Walker's Spicy Brussels Sprouts   231

Turkey Burgers with Guac Salsa   233

Curry Lentil Loaf   234

Raw Sunshine Wraps   236

Amy's Tempeh Chili   239

Roasted Lemon Asparagus with Pecans   241

Rawlicious Zucchini Pasta with Hemp Spinach Pesto   243

Mashed Cauliflower with Goat Cheese   244

Arugula or Kale Walnut Pesto   245

Sun-Dried Tomato Arugula Spelt Crust Pizza   246

Spaghetti Squash with Chia Seeds   248

Curry Chicken Burgers with Mango Salsa or Tzatziki

The spices make these juicy burgers incredibly flavorful. Enjoy them with a few spoonfuls of mango salsa or tzatziki. They're great as a power-packed lunch with a big raw salad and your favorite dressing the next day.

Makes 4 to 6 burgers

 Gluten-free

Burgers

1 lb (450 g) ground organic chicken breast

3 shallots, finely chopped

1 tbsp (15 mL) curry powder

1 tbsp (15 mL) lemon juice

1 tsp (5 mL) ground ginger

1 tsp (5 mL) ground cumin

¼ tsp (1 mL) cayenne pepper

Salt and black pepper

Mango Salsa

2 mangoes, peeled and thinly sliced

½ small red onion, thinly sliced

1 green onion, finely chopped

½ cup (125 mL) chopped cilantro

¼ cup (60 mL) lime juice

Tzatziki

½ cucumber, grated

1 to 2 cloves garlic

¾ cup (175 mL) sheep's milk yogurt

1 tbsp (15 mL) lemon juice

For the burgers, in a large bowl, combine all ingredients. Gently mix with your hands. Form into 4 to 6 patties, depending on how large you like your burgers. Cover and refrigerate for at least 20 minutes to let the flavors mingle.

Meanwhile, make the salsa or tzatziki. Combine all the salsa ingredients in a small bowl. Or, place all the tzatziki ingredients in a food processor and blend until smooth.

Preheat grill to medium.

Grill burgers until no pink is visible inside and juices run clear, 7 to 8 minutes per side. Top burgers with mango salsa or tzatziki.

Baked Lemon Pepper Salmon with "Cream" Sauce

This lemon-infused salmon is bright and fresh, just perfect for a cold winter's day. The creamy tahini dressing is a wonderful dairy-free alternative. Enjoy with Tamari Broccoli (page 230) and you'll have a well-balanced, joyous meal!

Serves 2

 DF Dairy-free   **GF** Gluten-free   **J** Joyous Comfort

2 salmon fillets, 6 oz (170 g) each
Juice of ½ lemon
Sea salt and freshly ground pepper

Lemon Pepper Tahini Sauce

2 tbsp (30 mL) extra-virgin olive oil
Grated zest and juice of 1 lemon
¼ cup (60 mL) tahini
1 tbsp (15 mL) honey
A sprinkle or two of sea salt and lots of
    freshly ground pepper

Preheat oven to 350°F (180°C).

Place salmon fillets on a baking sheet. Drizzle salmon with lemon juice and season with sea salt and black pepper. Bake for 10 to 15 minutes or until the inside of the fish is no longer dark pink.

Meanwhile, make the sauce. In a small bowl, stir together oil, lemon zest, lemon juice, tahini and honey. Season with sea salt and pepper.

Arrange baked salmon on plates and drizzle with sauce.

Joyous Tip

Tahini (also known as sesame paste) is a nutrient-dense paste made from ground sesame seeds. It is a good source of plant-based calcium. Some manufacturers add additional oils to their tahini—avoid those brands! Read your label to ensure there are no added oils. You want a tahini made only from pure ground sesame seeds to get the most nutritional bang for your buck.

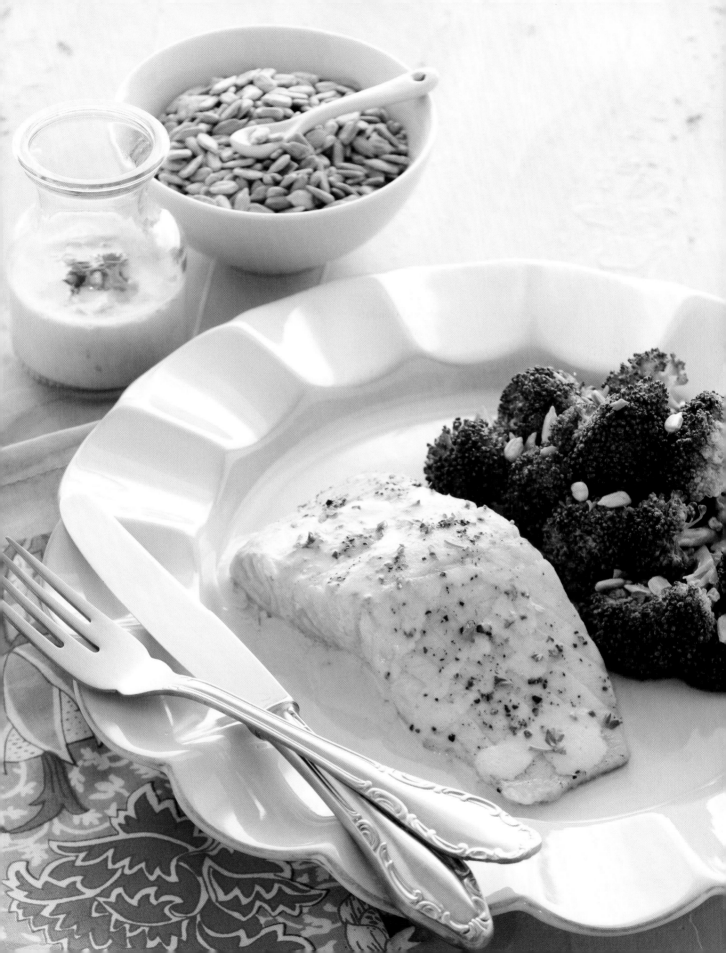

Tamari Broccoli with Sunflower Seeds

Fast-fresh-food is the best way to describe this side dish because it can be whipped up in no time to accompany any fish or chicken. The rich flavors in the tamari sauce add a memorable taste, and broccoli is a cancer-preventative power food.

Serves 2

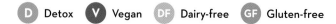

D Detox   **V** Vegan   **DF** Dairy-free   **GF** Gluten-free

2 tbsp (30 mL) coconut oil

1 bunch broccoli, cut in bite-size florets

1 to 2 tsp (5 to 10 mL) wheat-free tamari sauce

½ cup (125 mL) sunflower seeds

Melt coconut oil in a large saucepan over medium heat. Add broccoli and cook, stirring frequently, until bright green, 6 to 7 minutes. Drizzle with tamari and cook for another minute. Remove from heat and sprinkle with sunflower seeds.

Joyous Tip

Tamari is fermented soybean sauce with little or no wheat. It has a deeper, richer flavor than soy sauce—I prefer it. My favorite brand is San-J because it's made with 100 percent organic whole soybeans and no wheat. There is also a gluten-free tamari by this brand.

Walker's Spicy Brussels Sprouts

If your memories of Brussels sprouts make you crinkle your nose, you are not alone, but it's time to give this incredibly nutrient-dense anti-cancer food another chance! This recipe is one of my absolute favorites, especially when Walker, my hubs, makes it for me. These taste delicious chilled the next day!

Serves 2 generously

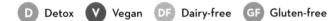 Detox   Vegan   Dairy-free   Gluten-free

2 tbsp (30 mL) coconut oil

2 cups (500 mL) Brussels sprouts, trimmed, cut in half

2 to 3 tsp (10 to 15 mL) hot chili flakes

½ tsp (2 mL) sea salt

Freshly ground pepper

In a large skillet, melt coconut oil over medium heat. Add Brussels sprouts and cook, stirring often, for 15 to 20 minutes or until tender. If the pan gets dry add some more coconut oil or 2 tbsp (30 mL) filtered water. Near the end of the cooking time, stir in chili flakes, salt and pepper.

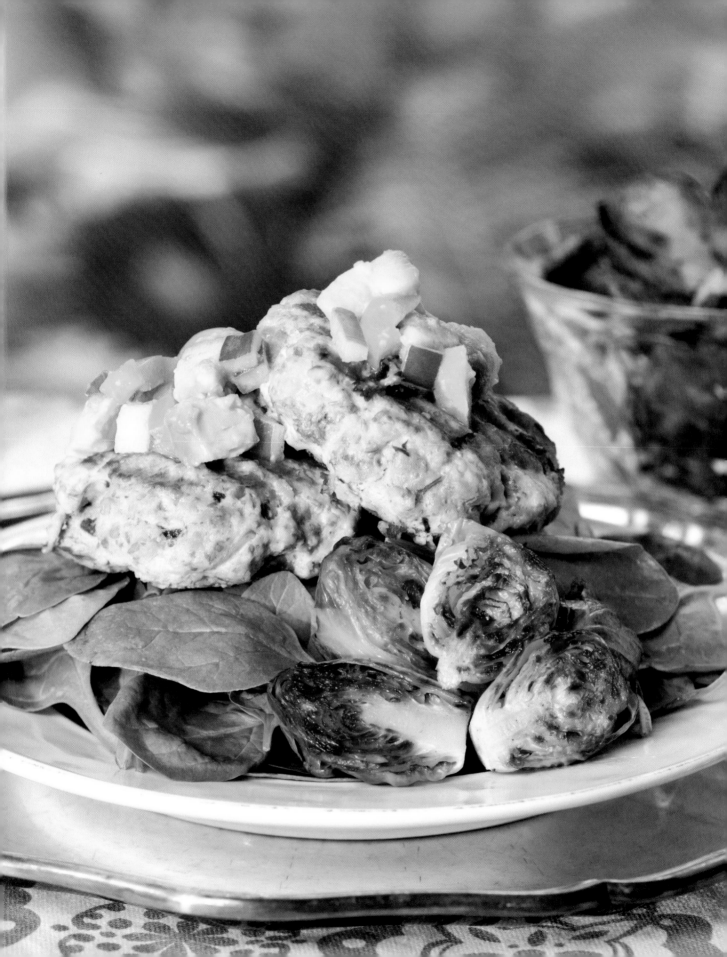

Turkey Burgers with Guac Salsa

This recipe is fabulous any time of year—it's fresh and light for the warmer months, but the flavors are rich and comforting for winter. I love making extra burgers and eating them chilled the next day with a salad—so satisfying! I love homemade salsa and guacamole, so I combined them in this fresh, vibrant topping for the burgers.

Makes 4 to 6 burgers

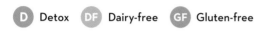 **D** Detox **DF** Dairy-free **GF** Gluten-free

Guac Salsa

2 ripe avocados, peeled and cubed

1 tomato, chopped

½ small red onion, finely chopped

1 clove garlic, minced

Juice of 1 to 2 limes

Pinch of sea salt

Burgers

1 egg (or 1 tbsp/15 mL chia seeds soaked in ¼ cup/60 mL water for 4 minutes)

2 tbsp (30 mL) wheat-free tamari sauce

1 lb (450 g) ground organic turkey

1 sweet onion, chopped

1 clove garlic, chopped

8 sun-dried tomatoes, sliced in slivers

5 to 7 cremini mushrooms, chopped

¼ cup (60 mL) chopped fresh parsley

1 tbsp (15 mL) hot chili flakes

Preheat grill to medium or oven to 350°F (180°C).

For the guac salsa, in a small bowl, combine avocados, tomato, onion and garlic; stir. Pour lime juice to taste over top and sprinkle with sea salt. Set aside.

For the burgers, in a large bowl, whisk together egg and tamari. Add turkey, onion, garlic, tomatoes, mushrooms, parsley and chili flakes; mix well with your hands (it's messy, so you might want to wear gloves). Form into 4 to 6 patties, depending on how large you like your burgers.

Grill burgers, with the lid closed and turning once, for 10 to 12 minutes or until cooked completely. Or bake for 7 to 9 minutes, flip them over and bake for another 7 to 9 minutes. Serve with Guac Salsa.

. . . .

Joyous Tip

I love these bun-free burgers with a side of Walker's Spicy Brussels Sprouts (page 231).

. . . .

Curry Lentil Loaf

This is a Joyous Health blog readers' favorite recipe and was a hit on my first online program, the Joyous 10-day online detox. The fiber-rich lentils make this recipe heart-healthy and detox-friendly. Perfect for making on a Sunday afternoon and enjoying for lunch during the week. It freezes really well too.

Serves 6 to 8

(D) Detox   (V) Vegetarian   (DF) Dairy-free   (GF) Gluten-free   (J) Joyous Comfort

¾ cups (175 mL) red or orange lentils

3½ cups (875 mL) filtered water

½ cup (125 mL) quinoa

2 tbsp (30 mL) coconut oil

1 small onion, chopped

1 cup (250 mL) sliced cremini mushrooms

½ cup (125 mL) finely chopped
   sweet red pepper

2 eggs (any size), lightly beaten

2 cloves garlic, minced

1 cup (250 mL) chopped fresh parsley
   or cilantro

¾ cup (175 mL) old-fashioned or
   quick-cooking rolled oats

½ cup (125 mL) pecans or almonds,
   coarsely chopped

3 tbsp (15 mL) curry powder

2 pinches of sea salt and lots of
   freshly ground pepper

Arugula or spinach

Preheat oven to 350°F (180°C). Grease a 13×9-inch (3 L) baking dish with coconut oil.

In a medium saucepan, bring lentils and 2½ cups (625 mL) of the water to a boil. Reduce heat and simmer, partly covered, just until tender, 15 to 25 minutes. Be careful not to overcook the lentils.

Meanwhile, in a separate small pot, bring quinoa and remaining 1 cup (250 mL) of water to a boil. Reduce heat and simmer, partly covered, until fluffy, about 15 minutes.

Meanwhile, melt coconut oil in a large saucepan over medium heat. Cook the onion, mushrooms and red pepper, stirring frequently, for 5 minutes or until tender.

In a large bowl, combine lentils, quinoa, mushroom mixture, eggs, garlic, parsley, oats, pecans, curry powder, salt and pepper to taste. Mix well with your hands. Transfer mixture to baking pan. Bake for 30 to 35 minutes or until golden brown. Serve this comforting loaf on a bed of peppery arugula or spinach.

. . . .

Joyous Tip

If you find the finished loaf a little crumbly, it's likely because you overcooked the lentils. Solution: Enjoy the loaf with a generous dollop of extra-virgin olive or hemp oil and a drizzle of balsamic vinegar on top.

. . . .

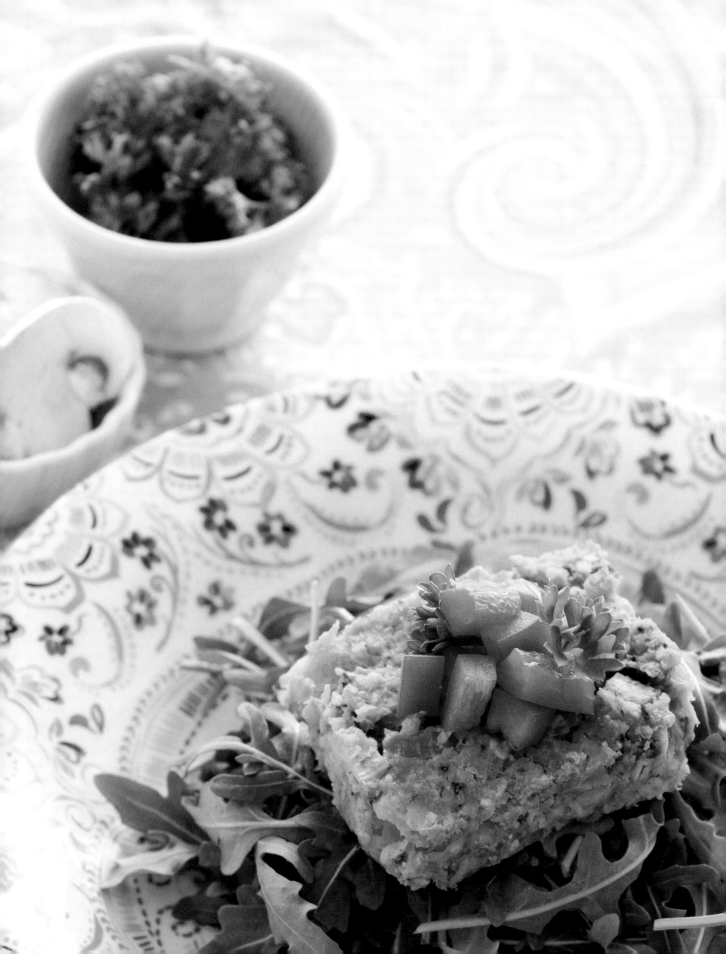

Raw Sunshine Wraps

You'll feel like a "raw foodie" when you eat these wraps. Because all the veggies are raw, these wraps are bursting with enzymes. Enzymes are the worker bees of every action in your body, from thinking to lifting your arm. You can eat 3 or 4 wraps as a meal or 1 or 2 as an energizing snack. The Thai-inspired almond sauce is zesty. Bring these to a party and they'll be a sure winner!

Makes 4 wraps

(D) Detox (V) Vegan (DF) Dairy-free (GF) Gluten-free (R) Raw

Almond Sauce

½ ripe avocado, peeled

1 clove garlic, minced

Juice of ½ lemon

1 tbsp (15 mL) almond butter

2 tsp (10 mL) grated fresh ginger

1 tsp (5 mL) wheat-free tamari sauce

⅓ cup (75 mL) filtered water

Wraps

4 collard greens or large kale leaves

½ cup (125 mL) thinly sliced purple cabbage

1 carrot, cut in matchsticks

2 green onions, cut in matchsticks

6 snow peas or green beans, thinly sliced lengthwise

1 cucumber, cut in matchsticks

1 avocado, peeled and sliced

Optional: pea shoots

For the almond sauce, place all the ingredients in a food processor and process until smooth. Set aside.

To assemble the wraps: With a knife, score the center rib of each collard green to make it easier to fold. In a bowl, toss together cabbage, carrot, green onions, snow peas and cucumber. Spread a dollop of almond sauce on the inside of each collard green. Place a small handful of vegetable mixture in the center of each collard green. Top with a slice or two of avocado and some pea shoots, if using. Roll up leaves like a wrap. You can roll from a narrow end or from the side—it's up to you. Insert a toothpick to secure, if needed. Use any leftover almond sauce as a dip. Sometimes I make double the almond sauce just for a dip.

. . . .

Joyous Tip

If you'd like to make the almond sauce more "hearty," add 2 tbsp (30 mL) hemp seeds for a complete source of protein and satiating good fat. In fact, hemp seeds are a wonderful source of a special kind of fatty acid called GLA, which is anti-inflammatory and can be beneficial for conditions such as arthritis and heart disease and for skin problems such as dermatitis.

You can use rice paper wraps instead of collard greens, but the wraps aren't raw.

. . . .

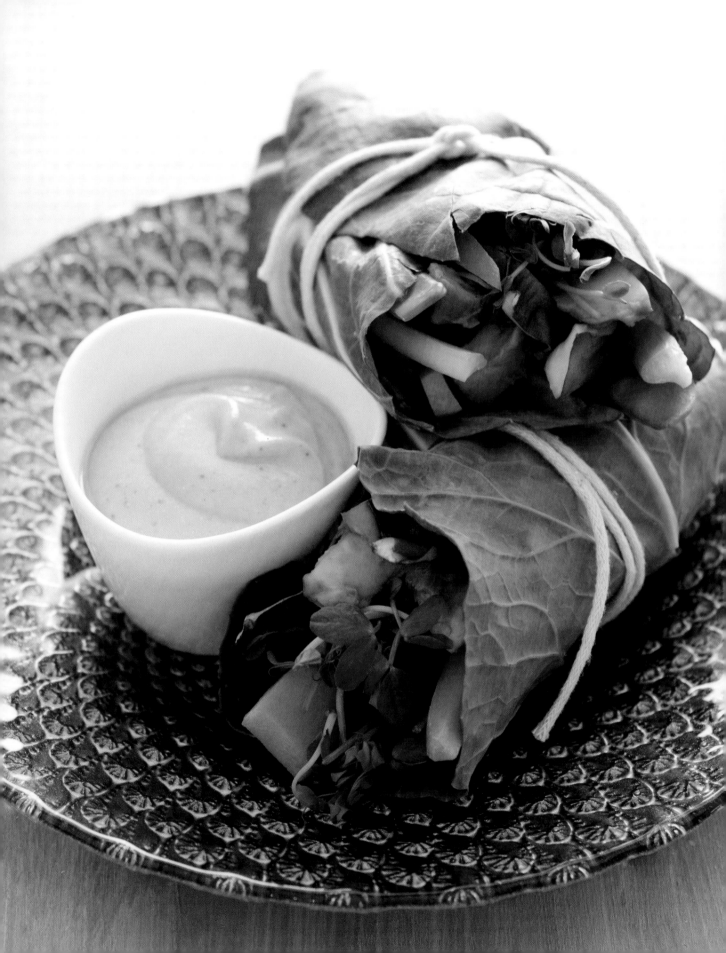

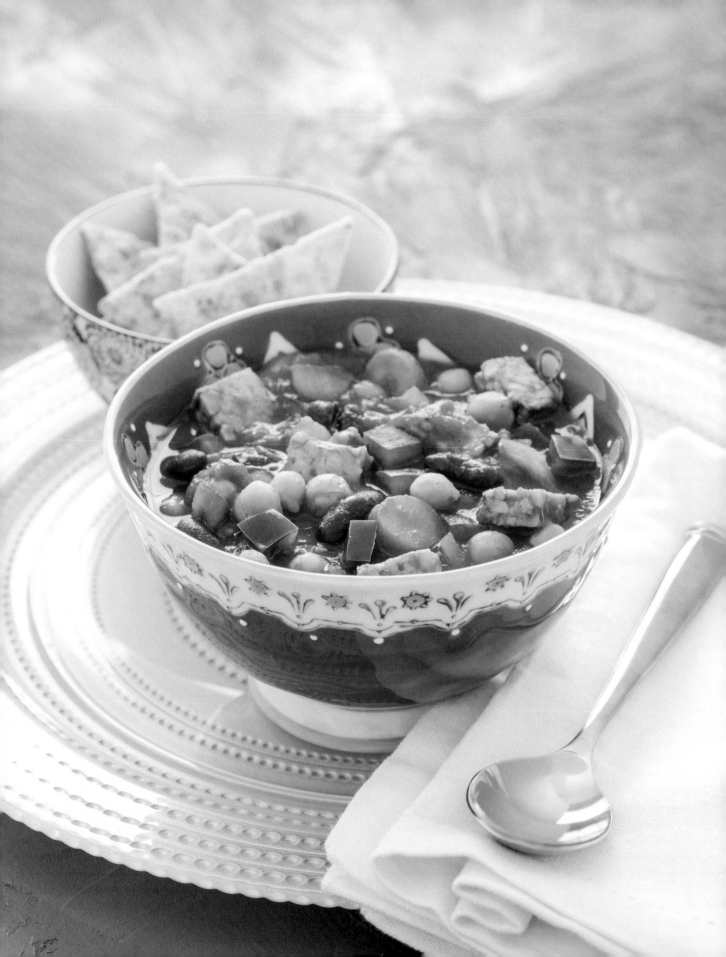

Amy's Tempeh Chili

My cousin Amy has been a vegetarian for as long as I can remember. When we were kids she was always served something intriguing at family Easter and Christmas celebrations instead of ham or turkey. The first time I made this recipe of hers for my hubby, Walker, he teased me, wondering how chili can possibly be tasty without ground beef. To his surprise he totally loved it, and now it's a regular dinner in our home—score!

Serves 4 to 6

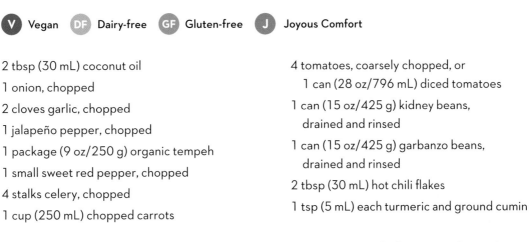 **V** Vegan   **DF** Dairy-free   **GF** Gluten-free   **J** Joyous Comfort

2 tbsp (30 mL) coconut oil

1 onion, chopped

2 cloves garlic, chopped

1 jalapeño pepper, chopped

1 package (9 oz/250 g) organic tempeh

1 small sweet red pepper, chopped

4 stalks celery, chopped

1 cup (250 mL) chopped carrots

4 tomatoes, coarsely chopped, or
     1 can (28 oz/796 mL) diced tomatoes

1 can (15 oz/425 g) kidney beans,
     drained and rinsed

1 can (15 oz/425 g) garbanzo beans,
     drained and rinsed

2 tbsp (30 mL) hot chili flakes

1 tsp (5 mL) each turmeric and ground cumin

Melt coconut oil in a large pot over medium heat. Add onion, garlic and jalapeño; cook, stirring frequently, for 5 minutes. Crumble three-quarters of the tempeh into the pot. Cook, stirring frequently, for 5 minutes. Add red pepper, celery and carrots; cook, stirring frequently, for 5 minutes. Add more coconut oil if necessary. Add tomatoes with their juice, kidney beans, garbanzo beans, chili flakes, turmeric and cumin. Increase heat and bring to a gentle boil, then reduce heat and simmer, stirring occasionally, for at least 30 minutes. Season with sea salt and pepper. Serve topped with crumbled remaining tempeh.

. . . .

Joyous Tip

My favorite brand of tempeh is Henry's because it's certified organic, non-GMO and a Canadian company from Kitchener-Waterloo, Ontario. Tempeh is a fermented soybean product. It's an excellent source of protein and is much easier to digest than tofu.

. . . .

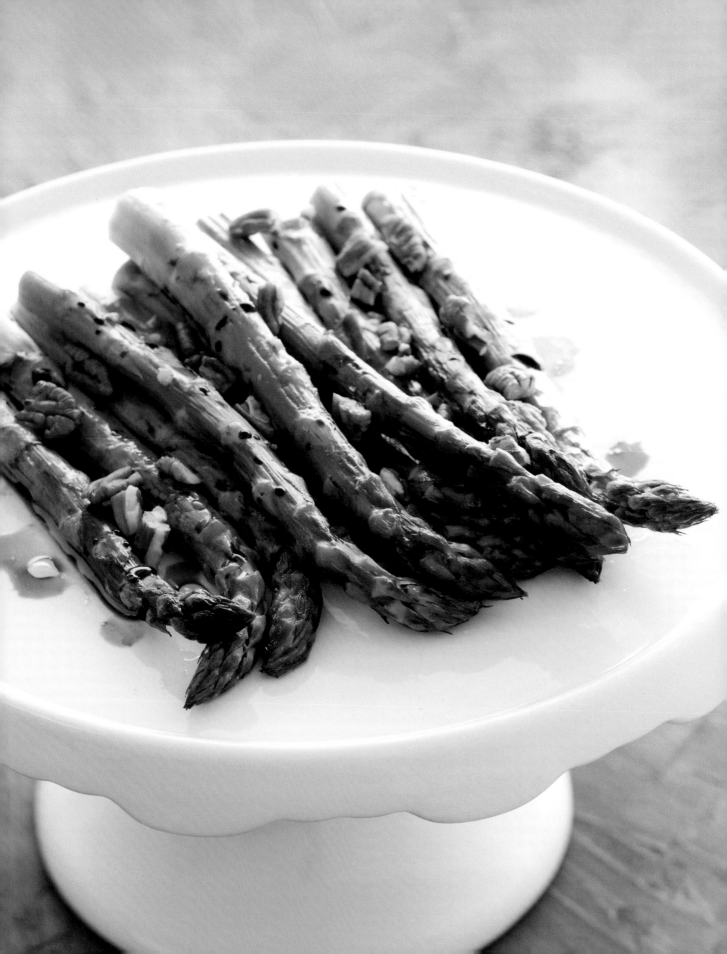

Roasted Lemon Asparagus with Pecans

Once spring hits, I can't help but smile because this means organic asparagus is in abundance at farmers' markets. This mouthwatering side dish is also wonderful served chilled for lunch.

Serves 4

D Detox **V** Vegan **DF** Dairy-free **GF** Gluten-free

1 lb (450 g) asparagus (preferably thick spears)

2 tbsp (30 mL) balsamic vinegar or juice of 1 lemon

1 to 2 tbsp (15 to 30 mL) grapeseed oil

2 pinches of sea salt and freshly ground black pepper

½ cup (125 mL) chopped pecans

Preheat oven to 350°F (180°C).

Snap tough ends off asparagus and discard. Place asparagus in a large baking dish or baking sheet. Sprinkle with balsamic or lemon juice and grapeseed oil and roll asparagus around to coat well. Season with sea salt and pepper.

Roast for 18 to 20 minutes or until fork-tender. Transfer to a platter and sprinkle with pecans.

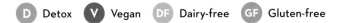

Joyous Tip

You may be surprised not to see extra-virgin olive oil in this recipe. This is because I do not recommend heating olive oil to a high temperature, as heat destroys the beneficial qualities of the oil. Grapeseed oil is the next best option for this recipe. You may drizzle high-quality extra-virgin olive oil (evoo) over the asparagus after it's been roasted to perfection. My favorite brand of evoo is from Acropolis Organics; www.acropolisorganics.com.

Asparagus is a source of a prebiotic fiber called inulin. Once inulin arrives in our large intestine, it becomes an ideal food source for certain types of bacteria associated with better nutrient absorption, lower risk of colon cancer and lower risk of allergies.

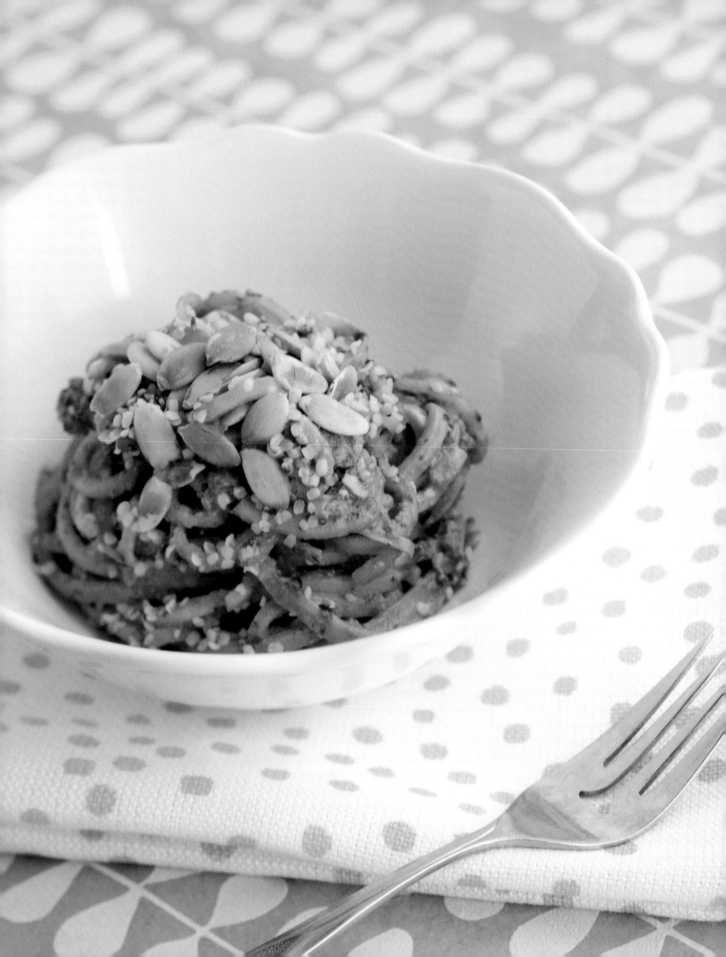

Rawlicious Zucchini Pasta with Hemp Spinach Pesto

This recipe is completely raw, hence "rawlicious." Raw recipes are chock-full of enzymes, vitamins and minerals. When I don't feel like turning on an oven, this is one of my go-tos, especially in the summer when zucchinis are growing like mad in Ma McCarthy's garden up north.

Serves 2

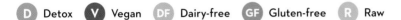

D Detox   **V** Vegan   **DF** Dairy-free   **GF** Gluten-free   **R** Raw

2 zucchinis, ends trimmed

Hemp Spinach Pesto

3 cups (750 mL) spinach

1 or 2 cloves garlic

½ cup (125 mL) pumpkin seeds

¼ cup (60 mL) hemp oil
   or extra-virgin olive oil

½ tsp (2 mL) sea salt

Optional: ½ cup (125 mL) hemp seeds

Use a spiralizer* to turn zucchinis into noodles, or use a vegetable peeler to slice zucchinis into ribbons. Place zucchini noodles in a large bowl.

For the pesto, in a food processor, combine all ingredients. Process to desired consistency. I personally like my pesto with a bit of texture, a little crunchy, but you can blend until creamy if you like. Add more oil if needed.

Add pesto to zucchini noodles and stir well.

*A spiralizer is a handy little gadget that turns zucchini into perfectly sized noodles. I like the Paderno brand. Make sure to include the skin, as it's full of fiber and nutrients.

Joyous Tip

Zucchini is high in a trace mineral called manganese, which helps the body metabolize protein and carbohydrates, participates in the production of sex hormones (ooh la la!) and catalyzes the synthesis of fatty acids and cholesterol.

Mashed Cauliflower with Goat Cheese

This creamy yet light side dish is the perfect replacement for mashed potatoes. Now, being a nutritionist, I would never bash a vegetable. However, white potatoes are not the best choice for a carb to accompany your meal, because they are not the most nutrient-dense vegetable. I promise you won't miss the potatoes here!

Serves 4

 D Detox   **V** Vegetarian   **GF** Gluten-fre   **J** Joyous Comfort

1 large cauliflower (2¾ lb/1.25 kg), stems and florets cut in bite-size pieces

½ cup (125 mL) soft goat cheese

1 tbsp (15 mL) almond milk

½ tsp (2 mL) salt

¼ tsp (1 mL) pepper

2 tbsp (30 mL) chopped fresh chives

In a steamer basket, cover and steam cauliflower until tender, about 10 minutes. Transfer to a large bowl.

Using a potato masher, mash cauliflower until the texture of mashed potatoes. Add goat cheese, almond milk, salt and pepper; stir until combined. Top with chives.

Arugula or Kale Walnut Pesto

If you enjoy garlic as much as I do, then you will love this pesto. It will become a favorite in your home because you can use it for pasta or on pizza, make salad dressing with it or enjoy it on crackers. Garlic has superfood status, and you can find it locally grown. The nice thing about this pesto is that you can use just about any leafy green, and you don't have to use pine nuts to call it "pesto"! Pine nuts can be very pricey, which is why I like using walnuts, almonds or cashews.

Makes about ¾ cup (175 mL)

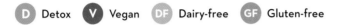

(D) Detox   (V) Vegan   (DF) Dairy-free   (GF) Gluten-free

2 cups (500 mL) arugula or baby spinach
   (or 5 or 6 kale leaves, washed and patted dry)
½ to 1 clove garlic
   (go easy on the garlic if you are a newbie to this recipe!)
½ cup (125 mL) walnuts, almonds or cashews
Juice of ½ lemon
¼ cup (60 mL) extra-virgin olive oil
Pinch of sea salt

If using kale, tear it away from the tough stems and tear into large pieces. Place all the ingredients in a food processor or high-powered blender; chop on high for 30 seconds to 1 minute. If you have a mini food processor, work in batches. Give it a taste test and add whatever ingredients you feel it needs. I usually add more oil.

Joyous Tip

Worried about the potent garlic smell on your breath? Chew on some parsley afterwards—it helps to neutralize the smell, plus it's a great source of calcium and a rich source of antioxidant nutrients such as vitamin C.

Sun-Dried Tomato Arugula Spelt Crust Pizza

Think you can't eat pizza because it's not healthy? Think again! When you use all real, "whole" ingredients, you can eat your pizza and enjoy it too. My good friend Dee, who transformed herself from a frozen-dinner girl to a kitchen goddess, made this pizza crust with her favorite toppings for me one night and I loved it. She's a pizza lover too.

Serves 2 to 3

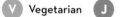 **V** Vegetarian **J** Joyous Comfort

Pizza Crust

1½ cups (375 mL) organic stone-ground
   spelt flour

1 tsp (5 mL) aluminum-free baking powder

½ tsp (2 mL) fine sea salt

1 egg (any size)

¼ cup (60 mL) water or almond milk

4 tbsp (60 mL) extra-virgin olive oil

Toppings

½ cup (125 mL) Arugula or
   Kale Walnut Pesto (page 245)

8 sun-dried tomatoes

½ cup (125 mL) soft goat cheese

½ cup (125 mL) fresh basil leaves

2 tbsp (30 mL) extra-virgin olive oil

Optional: 1 tsp (5 mL) hot chili flakes

Preheat oven to 425°F (220°C) with a pizza stone. Lightly oil a pizza pan or baking sheet.

For the pizza crust, in a medium bowl, stir together flour, baking powder and salt. In a small bowl, beat egg with a fork; stir in water and 2 tbsp (30 mL) of the olive oil. Add wet ingredients to dry ingredients and stir until they form a ball of dough. (A stand mixer with the dough hook will make it easier.) You may need to sprinkle the mixture with more flour to prevent it from sticking to the side of the bowl.

Lightly flour your work surface. Shape the dough into a ball. Knead it for 3 to 4 minutes or until smooth. (Or knead for 2 to 3 minutes in your stand mixer.) Using a floured rolling pin, roll dough into a circle slightly larger than your pizza stone or pizza pan or baking sheet. Scoop the rolled dough onto the pan. Using your hands, flatten it and press it to the edges. Brush dough with the remaining 2 tbsp (30 mL) oil. This will prevent the toppings from baking into the crust.

Top the pizza with as much arugula pesto as you like. Top with sun-dried tomatoes, goat cheese and basil. Bake for 20 minutes or until the edges are golden. Drizzle with extra-virgin olive oil and sprinkle with chili flakes if you like a little spice.

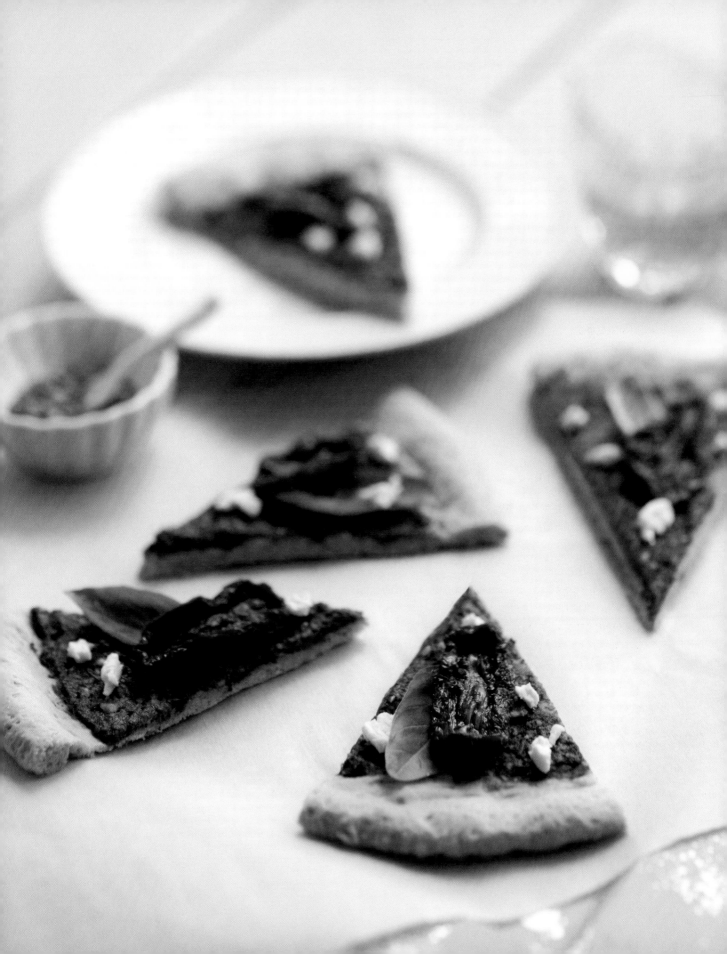

Spaghetti Squash with Chia Seeds

This can be a side dish or the main event used just like pasta. It's gluten-free, anti-belly-bloat and full of flavor. You can use this as a noodle and pour tomato sauce on top; you won't miss pasta one bit!

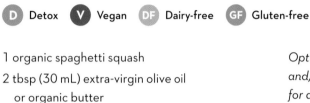

D Detox   **V** Vegan   **DF** Dairy-free   **GF** Gluten-free

1 organic spaghetti squash

2 tbsp (30 mL) extra-virgin olive oil or organic butter

½ tsp (2 mL) sea salt

Pinch of freshly ground pepper

2 tbsp (30 mL) chia seeds

½ cup (125 mL) chopped fresh parsley

Optional: 2 tbsp (30 mL) black sesame seeds and/or a sprinkle of organic nutritional yeast for a cheesy flavor

Preheat oven to 375°F (190°C).

Cut squash in half and scrape out all the seeds. Place the squash cut side down in a baking dish; add 1 inch (2.5 cm) filtered water. Bake, uncovered, for 50 minutes. Poke with a fork; if it is not tender, cook for 10 to 15 minutes longer or until fork-tender. Using a fork, scrape squash flesh into a serving bowl. It will be stringy like spaghetti and come out very easily.

Pour oil over squash and season with sea salt and pepper. Sprinkle with chia seeds and garnish with parsley. Add sesame seeds and organic nutritional yeast, if using.

. . . .

Joyous Tip

Separate the squash seeds from the stringy flesh, spread them on a baking sheet, sprinkle with sea salt and bake them at 225°F (110°C) for about 1½ hours. Enjoy as a snack!

Even though spaghetti squash is not on the "Dirty Dozen," make sure you buy organic squash, especially if you are pregnant or breast-feeding, as it tends to absorb from the soil a banned insecticide called dieldrin, which is still persistent in the environment.

. . . .

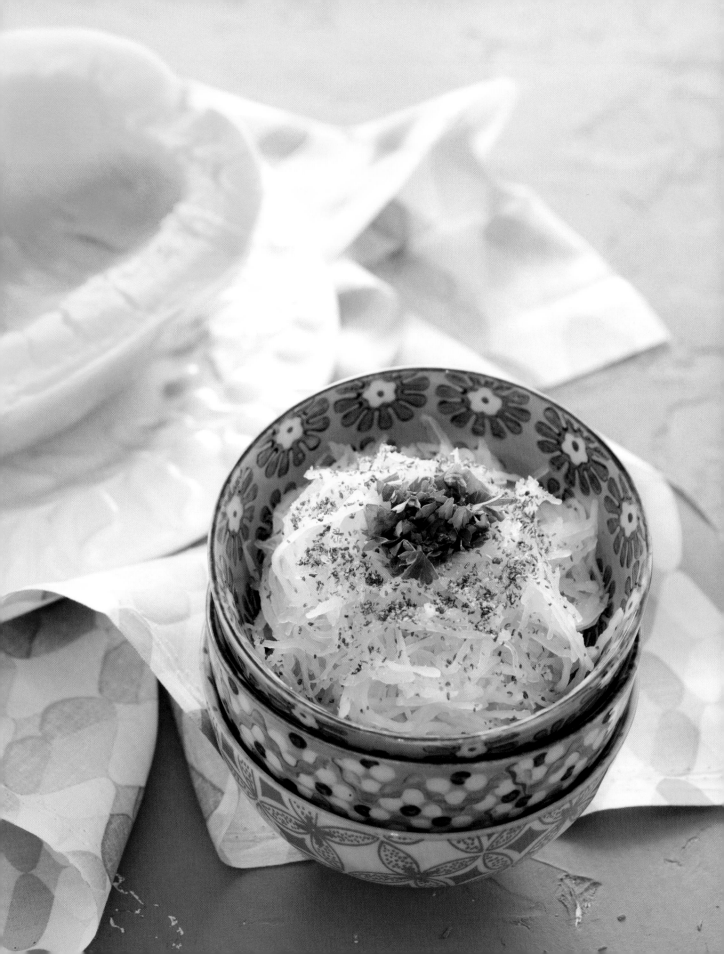

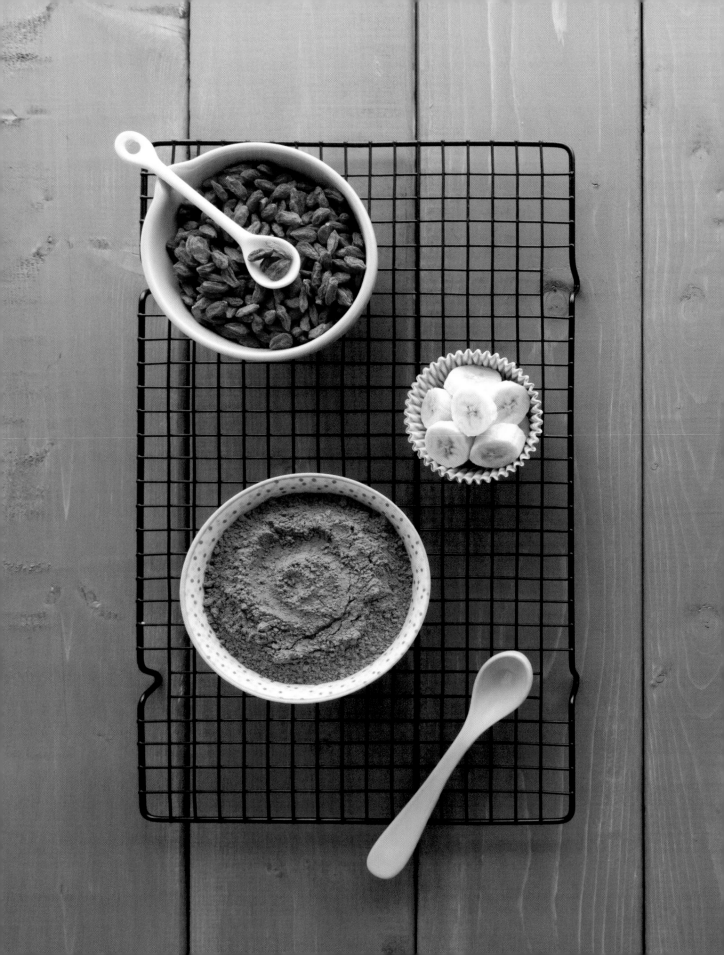

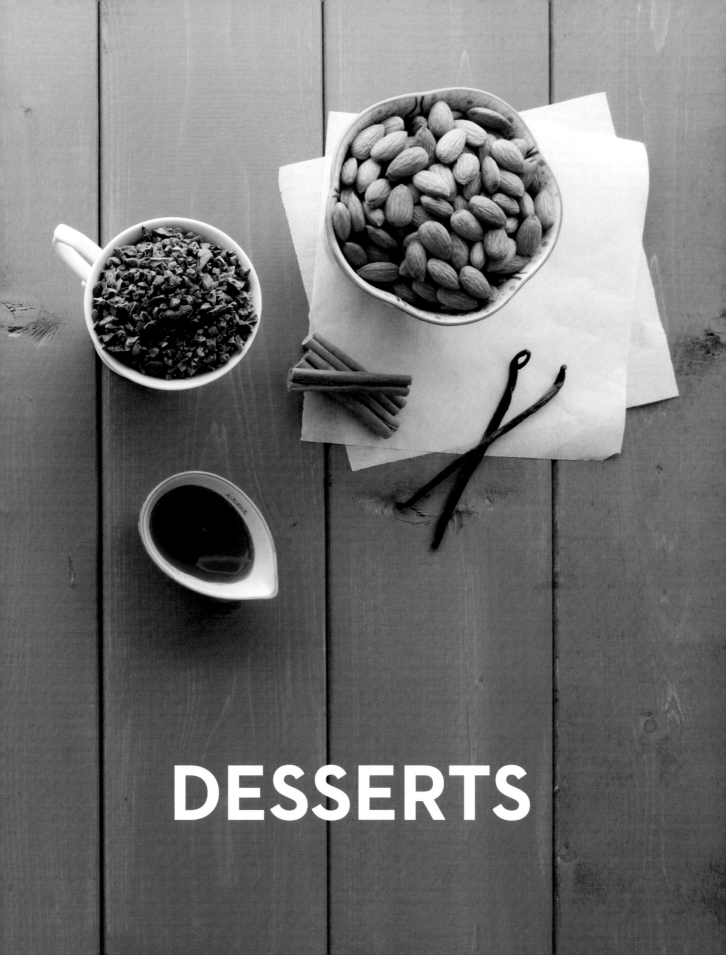

DESSERTS

Cardamom Apple Crisp   253

Fruit Salad with Cashew Orange Cream   254

Raspberry Maca Popsicles   257

Avocado Matcha Popsicles   257

Peaches and Cream Popsicles   258

Raw Carrot Cake Balls   258

Sexy Maca Balls   261

Double Chocolate Gluten-Free Cookies   262

Mom's Trail Mix Cookies   263

Chili and Cinnamon Chocolate Bark   264

Black Bean Chia Brownies   267

Lemon Poppy Seed Loaf with Coconut Icing   268

Chocolate Mint Pudding   270

Key Lime Pudding   271

Pear Tart with Cashew Maple Cream   273

Cardamom Apple Crisp

I created this dessert for some vegan friends I was hosting for dinner, so it's completely dairy-free (most crisps use butter in the topping). The cardamom was such a nice change from the usual cinnamon.

Serves 6 or 7

V Vegan   **DF** Dairy-free   **GF** Gluten-free   **J** Joyous Comfort

Topping

1½ cups (375 mL) quinoa flakes (pre-cooked)

2 tsp (10 mL) cinnamon

¼ tsp (1.25 mL) ground cardamom

¼ cup (60 mL) sulfite-free dried cranberries

¼ cup (60 mL) chopped pecans or walnuts

¼ cup (60 mL) coconut oil, melted

1 tbsp (15 mL) coconut sugar

1 to 2 tbsp (15 to 30 mL) real maple syrup

Filling

6 apples (unpeeled), washed, cored and thinly sliced

2 tbsp (30 mL) apple juice or water

1 tsp (5 mL) cinnamon

1 tbsp (15 mL) coconut sugar

Preheat oven to 350°F (180°C).

For the topping, in a medium bowl, stir together quinoa flakes, cinnamon and cardamom. Stir in cranberries, pecans, coconut oil and coconut sugar. Hold off on the maple syrup for now.

For the filling, in a large bowl, combine apples, apple juice and cinnamon; toss well. Taste one of the apples. If you want a sweeter filling, stir in the coconut sugar.

Transfer apples to a baking dish—you may use a deep round baking dish or a 13×9-inch (3 L) baking pan, depending on how thick you like the topping. Sprinkle topping evenly over apples; drizzle with maple syrup. Bake for 35 minutes or until apples are tender. I like my apples to have a little texture, so you may wish to bake for longer. Serve with coconut milk vanilla ice cream, or for breakfast with coconut milk.

. . . .

Joyous Tip

You will find pre-cooked quinoa flakes at most health food stores. They look like oat flakes and have a mild flavor. My favorite brand is GoGo Quinoa. If you can't find them, substitute with quick-cooking rolled oats.

. . . .

Fruit Salad with Cashew Orange Cream

This fruit salad is decadent with the cashew orange cream but completely guilt-free! Enjoy as a dessert or an afternoon snack.

Serves 4

(D) Detox (V) Vegan (DF) Dairy-free (GF) Gluten-free

1 pint (500 mL) strawberries, sliced in half

4 kiwifruit, peeled and cut in bite-size chunks

1 pint (500 mL) blueberries or blackberries

1 pineapple, peeled and cut in bite-size chunks

2 large oranges, segmented

Juice of 2 limes

Cashew Orange Cream

1 cup (250 mL) raw cashews
  (soaked for 4 hours and drained)

3 tbsp (45 mL) coconut milk

2 tbsp (30 mL) real maple syrup

1 tbsp (15 mL) grated orange zest

Juice from 1 freshly squeezed orange

In a large bowl, toss fruit with lime juice.

For the cashew orange cream, in a food processor or blender, combine all ingredients. Process until smooth like cream. Add more coconut milk if you prefer a thinner consistency.

Half-fill 4 dessert bowls with fruit. Add a heaping spoonful of cashew orange cream. Fill bowls with remaining fruit. Top with some more cream.

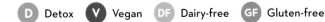

Joyous Tip

Many times I say to my clients, eat the food you want to look like! This tip applies here perfectly. Fruit is *full* of phytonutrients that lend them their beautiful rich colors. Many of these same nutrients are very beautifying for your skin. Plus there's a dose of vitamin C, which is a precursor to collagen and what your skin is literally made of.

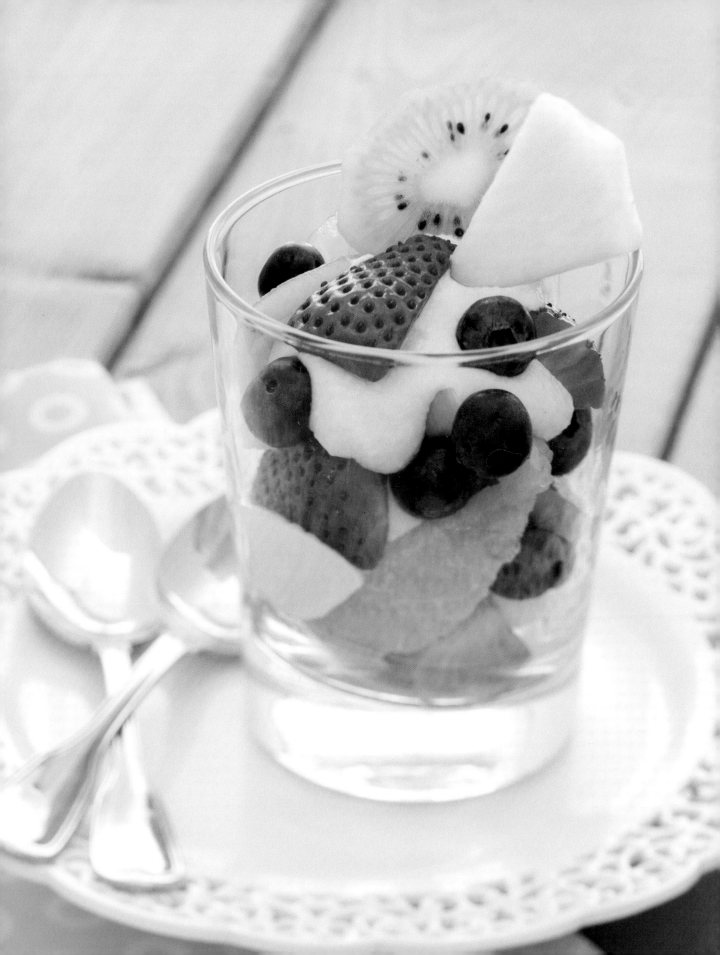

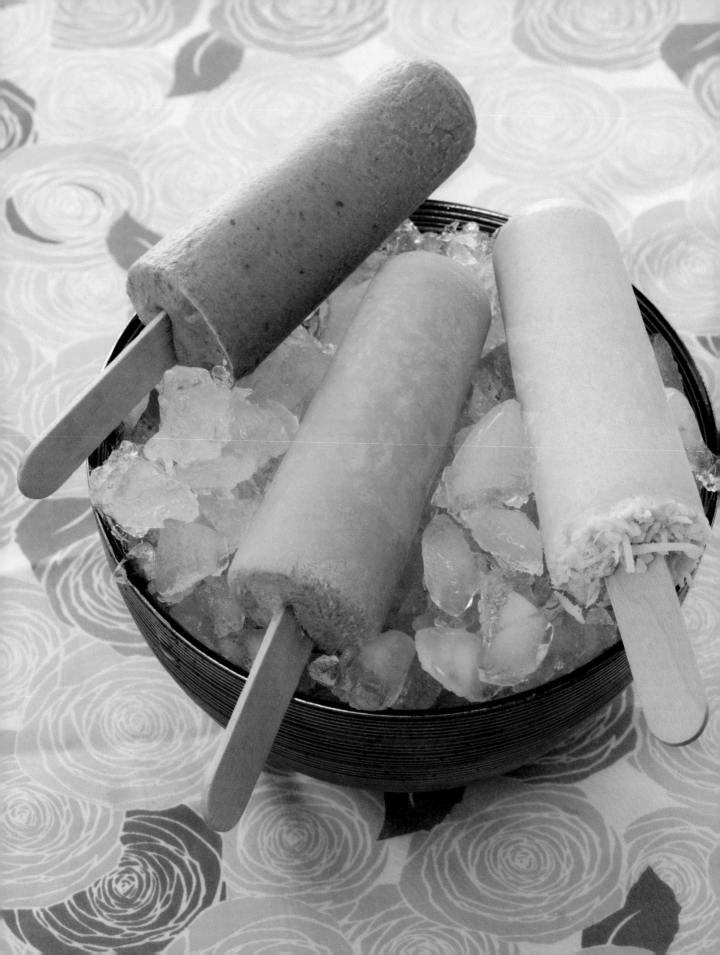

Perfect Popsicles Three Ways

When the heat of the summer hits, these wonderfully nourishing popsicles will cool you off like a cucumber. I've even snuck a few superfoods into each recipe! They are naturally sweet, but you can taste-test them before you pop them in the freezer and add more sweetness if you so desire. Each recipe makes 4 to 6 popsicles, depending on the size of your mold.

Raspberry Maca Popsicles

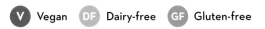 **Vegan**   **DF Dairy-free**   **GF Gluten-free**

1 can (14 oz/400 mL) coconut milk
2 pints (1 L) raspberries, washed
3 tbsp (45 mL) maca powder
3 tbsp (45 mL) chia seeds

3 tbsp (45 mL) almond butter
10 to 15 drops liquid stevia
 (or ½ cup/125 mL real maple syrup)

Shake can of coconut milk until you hear the milk change from solid to liquid. Place all ingredients in a blender or food processor; process until well combined. Pour into popsicle molds and freeze for at least 6 hours or overnight. If you have trouble removing the popsicles, run the mold under lukewarm water.

Joyous Tip

After washing raspberries, place them on a kitchen towel to dry off. You don't want excess water in the popsicles because it can cause freezer burn.

Avocado Matcha Popsicles

 Vegan   **DF Dairy-free**   **GF Gluten-free**

1 can (14 oz/400 mL) coconut milk
1 ripe medium avocado, peeled and cubed
1 tbsp (15 mL) matcha green tea powder

¼ cup (60 mL) honey
10 to 15 drops liquid stevia

Shake can of coconut milk until you hear the milk change from solid to liquid. Place all ingredients in a blender or food processor; process until well combined. Pour into popsicle molds and freeze for at least 6 hours or overnight. If you have trouble removing the popsicles, run the mold under lukewarm water.

Peaches and Cream Popsicles

 Vegan　 DF Dairy-free　 GF Gluten-free　 J Joyous Comfort

1 can (14 oz/400 mL) coconut milk

8 to 10 ripe medium peaches,
　peeled and cut in wedges

10 to 15 drops liquid stevia
　(or ½ cup/125 mL real maple syrup)

½ cup (125 mL) unsweetened sulfite-free
　coconut flakes

Shake can of coconut milk until you hear the milk change from solid to liquid. Place all ingredients, excluding coconut flakes, in a blender or food processor; process until well combined. Pour into popsicle molds. Sprinkle with coconut flakes. Freeze for at least 6 hours or overnight. If you have trouble removing the popsicles, run the mold under lukewarm water.

Raw Carrot Cake Balls

One of my all-time favorite desserts is carrot cake. These yummy cookie balls, made with shredded carrots and spices, taste just like it! Because they are completely raw, you can make them in a snap.

Makes 18 to 20 balls

V Vegetarian　 DF Dairy-free　 R Raw　 J Joyous Comfort

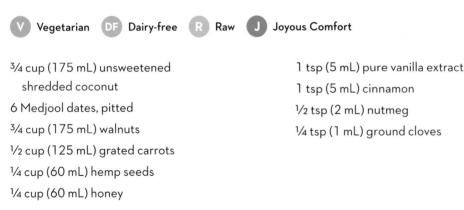

¾ cup (175 mL) unsweetened
　shredded coconut

6 Medjool dates, pitted

¾ cup (175 mL) walnuts

½ cup (125 mL) grated carrots

¼ cup (60 mL) hemp seeds

¼ cup (60 mL) honey

1 tsp (5 mL) pure vanilla extract

1 tsp (5 mL) cinnamon

½ tsp (2 mL) nutmeg

¼ tsp (1 mL) ground cloves

Reserve ¼ cup (60 mL) shredded coconut in a shallow dish for rolling. Place remaining ingredients in a high-powered food processor and process until fully combined. Form mixture into 1-inch (2.5 cm) balls and roll in reserved shredded coconut, coating balls completely. Transfer to a baking sheet and refrigerate for a few hours or overnight. Keep chilled, or freeze in an airtight container for a few months (though I guarantee they won't last that long). Enjoy 1 or 2 as a snack or dessert.

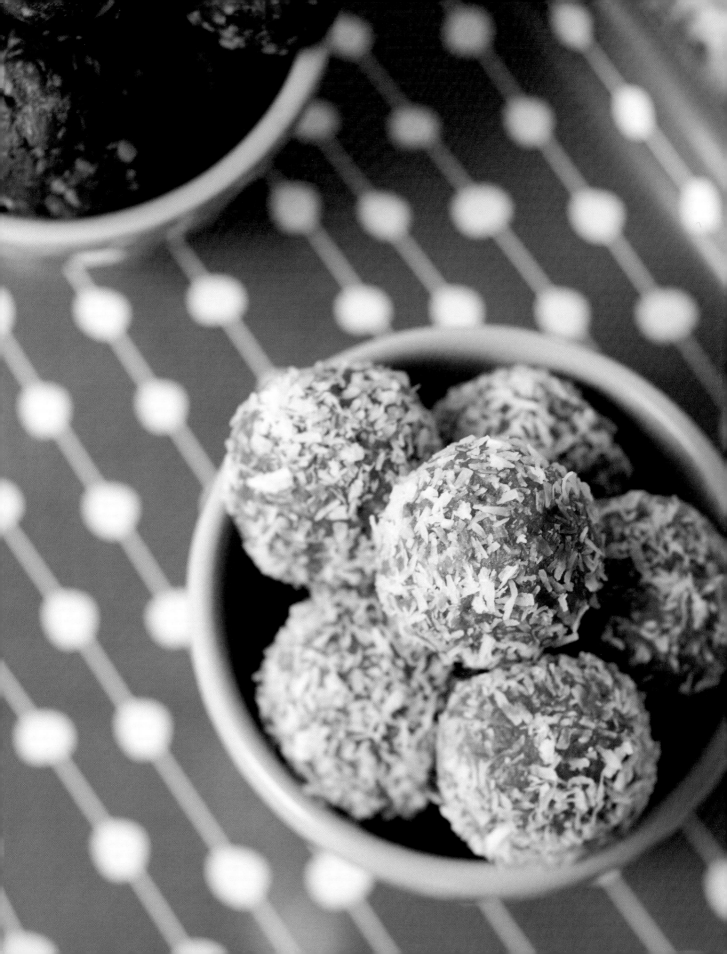

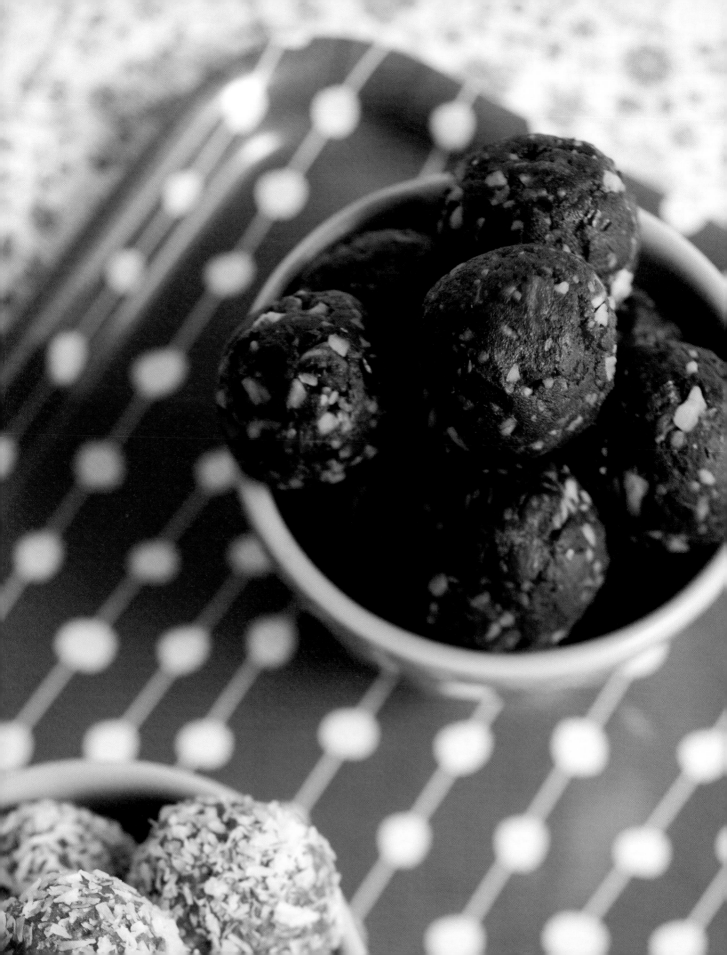

Sexy Maca Balls

This recipe is a Joyous Health blog readers' favorite because of the famous superfood maca—and maybe even a little because of the name. Maca is a Peruvian root reported to increase stamina and energy and help the body better adapt to stress. Ancient rumors have it that maca may even increase libido—ooh la la! These balls of deliciousness are the perfect sweet snack, with protein and good fat to fill the hunger gap mid-morning or mid-afternoon.

Makes 15 to 20 balls

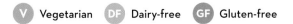 **V** Vegetarian **DF** Dairy-free **GF** Gluten-free

8 to 10 soft Medjool dates, pitted

½ cup (125 mL) raw almonds or cashews

¼ cup (60 mL) goji berries

¼ cup (60 mL) dark chocolate chips* or raw cacao nibs

1 tbsp (15 mL) cinnamon

1 tbsp (15 mL) raw cacao powder

1½ tsp (7 mL) maca powder

1 tsp (5 mL) pure vanilla extract

Place all ingredients in a high-powered food processor and process until combined. Roll mixture into 1-inch (2.5 cm) balls with your hands. Place on a baking sheet and refrigerate for a few hours or overnight. Keep chilled, or freeze in an airtight container for a few months (though I guarantee they won't last that long). Enjoy 1 or 2 as a snack or dessert.

Check ingredients label to confirm gluten-free if you want this recipe to be truly free of gluten.

Double Chocolate Gluten-Free Cookies

When I was experimenting in my kitchen one day I created these cookies. They are a chocolate lover's dream because of the double hit of chocolate from the raw cacao and cacao nibs. The coconut flour keeps them surprisingly moist. They're perfect with a glass of almond milk.

Makes 20 to 24 cookies

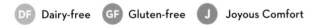 **DF** Dairy-free   **GF** Gluten-free   **J** Joyous Comfort

½ cup (125 mL) coconut flour

⅓ cup (75 mL) raw cacao powder

¼ cup (60 mL) coconut sugar

1 tsp (5 mL) baking powder

2 eggs (any size)

1 cup (250 mL) water or almond or hemp milk

1 tbsp (15 mL) coconut nectar or real maple syrup

1 tsp (5 mL) pure vanilla extract

¼ cup (60 mL) coconut oil, melted and cooled slightly

½ cup (125 mL) chocolate chips* or cacao nibs

Preheat oven to 350°F (180°C). Grease a baking sheet or line with parchment paper.

In a large bowl, whisk together coconut flour, cacao powder, coconut sugar and baking powder. In a medium bowl, lightly beat the eggs; add water, coconut nectar, vanilla and coconut oil. Add wet ingredients to dry ingredients; stir until well combined. Fold in chocolate chips. Form dough into 1-inch (2.5 cm) balls and arrange ½ inch (1 cm) apart on baking sheet. Flatten slightly.

Bake for 12 minutes or until tops are dry. Let cool on cookie sheet for 10 minutes, then transfer to a rack to cool completely.

*Check ingredients label to confirm gluten-free if you want this recipe to be truly free of gluten.

Mom's Trail Mix Cookies

My mom makes these cookies for me nearly every time I visit her, and I always get a care package to take home. These cookies are great with a nice cup of hot green tea and your favorite book on a quiet Sunday afternoon, or as an afternoon power snack at work. Use your favorite trail mix; I like Bob's Red Mill Old Country Style Muesli.

Makes 20 to 24 cookies

V Vegetarian   **DF** Dairy-free   **J** Joyous Comfort

¾ cup (175 mL) spelt flour or stone-ground whole wheat flour

½ tsp (2 mL) baking soda

½ tsp (2 mL) sea salt

½ tsp (2 mL) cinnamon

1 egg (any size)

½ cup (125 mL) coconut oil, melted

½ cup (125 mL) coconut sugar or Sucanat

1 tsp (5 mL) pure vanilla extract

1 cup (250 mL) trail mix

½ cup (125 mL) chocolate chips

¼ cup (60 mL) cacao nibs

Preheat oven to 375°F (190°C). Lightly grease a cookie sheet.

In a medium bowl, whisk together flour, baking soda, salt and cinnamon. In a large bowl, beat the egg; whisk in coconut oil, coconut sugar and vanilla. Add to flour mixture and mix with a spatula until well combined. Stir in trail mix, chocolate chips and cacao nibs. Drop by teaspoonfuls about ½ inch (1 cm) apart on cookie sheet. Press down carefully with a lightly floured fork.

Bake for 10 to 12 minutes or until edges are golden brown. Let cool on the cookie sheet for about 5 minutes, then transfer to a rack to cool completely.

Chili and Cinnamon Chocolate Bark

This recipe reminds me of my favorite spicy hot chocolate from Soma Chocolatemaker in Toronto's Distillery District. The hint of cayenne will give your metabolism a little boost, and you'll love how easy it is to make.

Makes about 8 medium pieces

 Vegan **GF** Gluten-free

⅓ cup (75 mL) coconut oil

¾ cup (175 mL) raw cacao powder

¼ cup (60 mL) real maple syrup (add more if you like it sweeter)

1 tbsp (15 mL) cinnamon

1 tsp (5 mL) cayenne pepper

¼ cup (60 mL) raw cashews, coarsely chopped

In a small saucepan over low heat, melt coconut oil. Slowly stir in cacao and maple syrup. When fully combined, stir in cinnamon and cayenne. Remove from heat and let cool for a few minutes. Line a baking sheet with parchment paper. Pour chocolate mixture onto the paper and sprinkle with cashews. Refrigerate for 4 hours. Break into pieces. Store in the fridge for up to 1 week or freeze for a couple of months.

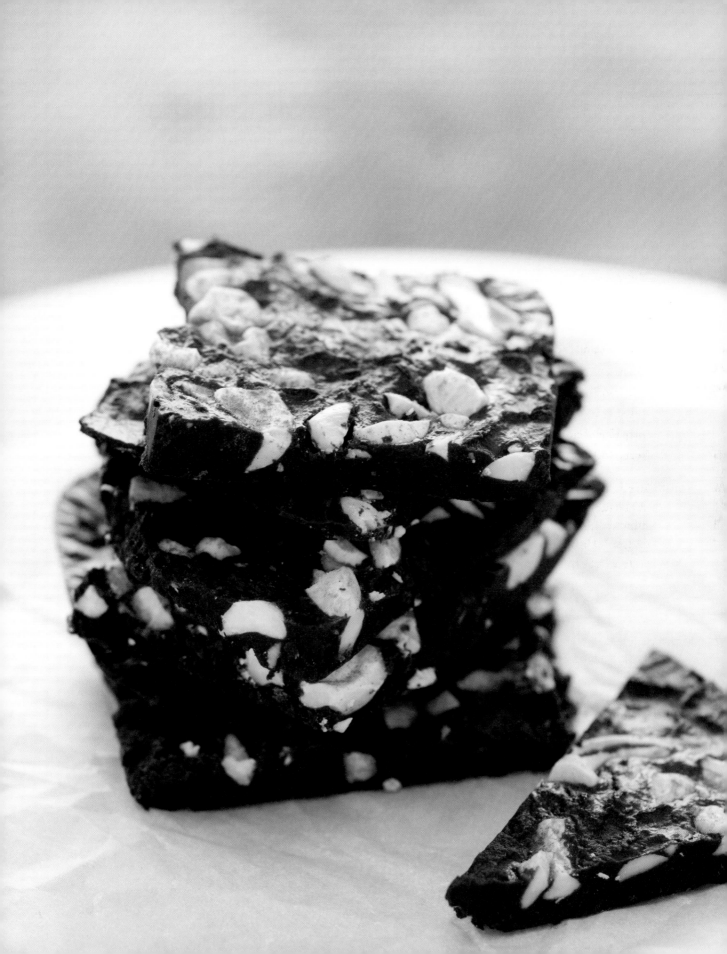

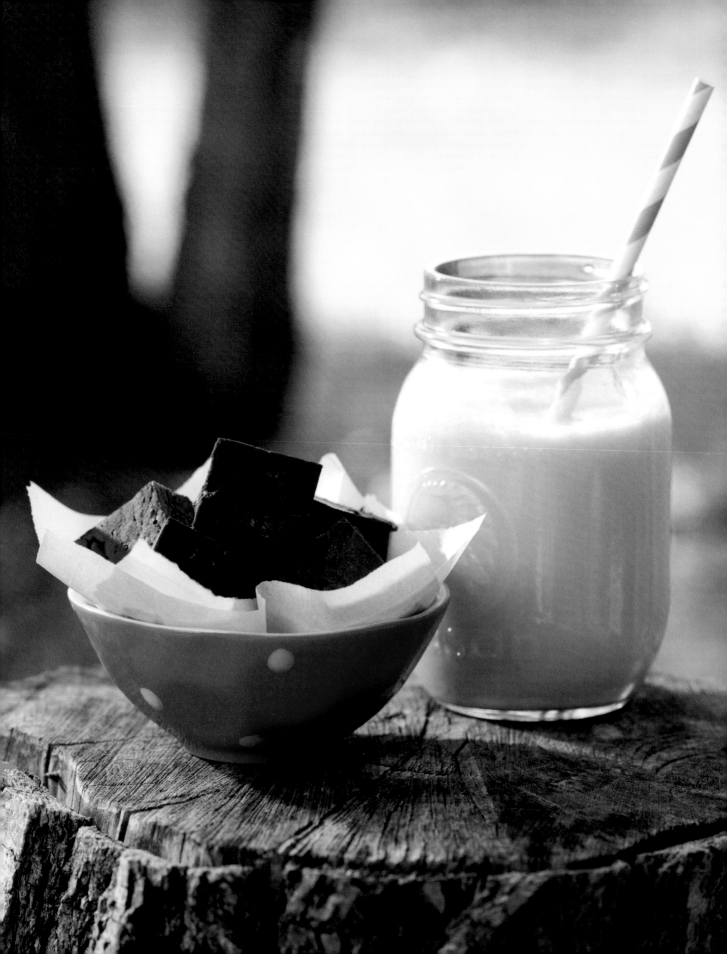

Black Bean Chia Brownies

Here is a much healthier version of regular brownies, but don't worry—you don't have to sacrifice flavor! And they are so delicious, no one will ever guess you've used black beans and chia seeds, infusing these brownies with tons of fiber. You could use regular cocoa powder, but it's just not as intensely flavorful—or nutrient-dense—as raw cacao powder. To make them gluten-free, choose GF chocolate chips.

Makes 24 small brownies

 Vegetarian 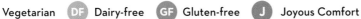 Dairy-free   GF Gluten-free   J Joyous Comfort

1 can (15 oz/425 g) black beans, drained and rinsed

3 medium eggs

½ cup (125 mL) coconut sugar

⅓ cup (75 mL) coconut oil, at room temperature

¼ cup (60 mL) raw cacao powder

2 tbsp (30 mL) chia seeds

2 tsp (10 mL) pure vanilla extract

½ cup (125 mL) semisweet dark chocolate chips

¼ cup (60 mL) raw cacao nibs

Preheat oven to 350°F (180°C). Grease an 8-inch (2 L) square baking pan.

In a food processor or blender, combine black beans, eggs, coconut sugar, coconut oil, cacao powder, chia seeds and vanilla. Process until smooth. Stir in chocolate chips. Transfer mixture to the baking pan. Level with a spatula and sprinkle with cacao nibs. Bake for 30 to 35 minutes or until a fork inserted in the center comes out clean. Cool in the pan before cutting.

Lemon Poppy Seed Loaf with Coconut Icing

This is a "healthy recipe makeover" success story! The typical lemon poppy seed loaf contains far too much refined sugar. One day I created this for a girlfriend who loved the refined sugar (unhealthy) version from her local coffee shop. She never went back and now makes this recipe all the time. Oh and PS the icing is foodgasmic!

Makes 1 loaf or 12 muffins

(V) Vegetarian   (DF) Dairy-free   (J) Joyous Comfort

2 cups (500 mL) spelt flour

½ cup (125 mL) coconut sugar

¼ cup (60 mL) poppy seeds

1 tsp (5 mL) baking powder

½ tsp (2 mL) baking soda

½ tsp (2 mL) sea salt

Grated zest and juice of 1 lemon

¼ cup (60 mL) grapeseed oil

½ cup (125 mL) almond milk

2 extra-large eggs, lightly beaten

Coconut Icing

½ cup (125 mL) coconut butter, at room temperature

¼ cup (60 mL) liquid honey

1 tsp (5 mL) pure vanilla extract

½ tsp (2 mL) grated lemon zest

Preheat oven to 350°F (180°C). Grease a loaf pan.

In a medium bowl, whisk together flour, sugar, poppy seeds, baking powder, baking soda, sea salt and lemon zest. Beating well after each addition, add grapeseed oil, almond milk, lemon juice and eggs.

Pour batter into loaf pan. Bake for 35 to 40 minutes or until a toothpick inserted in the center of the loaf comes out clean. Cool completely before applying icing. (I usually leave the loaf in the pan, cut out a slice, cover the loaf with plastic wrap and pop it back in the fridge.)

For the icing, combine all ingredients in a small bowl; stir until well combined. Enjoy immediately or refrigerate for a week.

Option: To make muffins, line a muffin pan with paper liners. Divide batter among muffin cups, filling three-quarters full. Bake for 22 to 24 minutes or until a toothpick inserted in the center of a muffin comes out clean. Cool completely before applying icing.

Joyous Tip

Coconut butter and coconut oil are not the same thing. Coconut butter is whole coconut flesh puréed into a fibrous, densely nutritious spread—think almond butter. Coconut oil is just that, the pure oil of the coconut, expressed much like peanut oil or olive oil. It's full of medium-chain triglycerides—very health-promoting fats. You do not need to store either in the refrigerator.

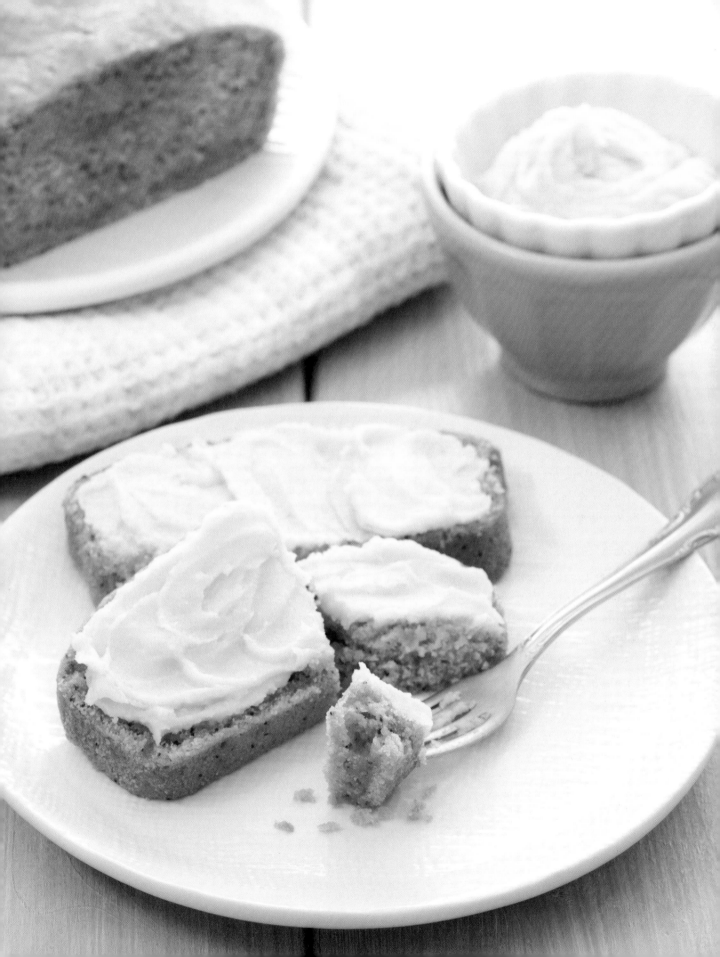

Chocolate Mint Pudding

Chocolate avocado pudding was one of first raw recipes I ever made for my blog. Because it was so popular, I created an orange version too. The chocolate mint idea came from Kate, my research assistant aka nutrition nerd at Joyous Health. If you've only ever had store-bought chocolate pudding, you are in for a real treat!

Serves 2 generously

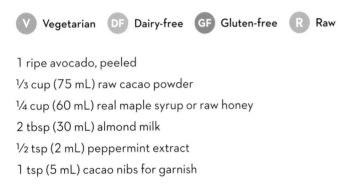

V Vegetarian   **DF** Dairy-free   **GF** Gluten-free   **R** Raw

1 ripe avocado, peeled
⅓ cup (75 mL) raw cacao powder
¼ cup (60 mL) real maple syrup or raw honey
2 tbsp (30 mL) almond milk
½ tsp (2 mL) peppermint extract
1 tsp (5 mL) cacao nibs for garnish

Place all ingredients except cacao nibs in a food processor or high-powered blender; process until nice and smooth. If you prefer a thinner consistency, add a little more almond milk and blend some more. Give it a taste test. If you prefer it sweeter, add more maple syrup or raw honey. Spoon into serving bowls and sprinkle with cacao nibs.

Joyous Tip

Simply Organic makes various organic flavored extracts. You can find them at most health food stores or in the health food section of your grocery store.

Key Lime Pudding

Two desserts I love are Key lime pie and any flavor of pudding, so I combined them into one fresh-tasting and completely raw (no-bake!) recipe. This dessert is proof that healthy and delicious can be found in the same recipe.

Serves 4

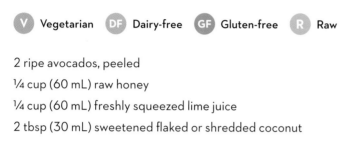

V Vegetarian **DF** Dairy-free **GF** Gluten-free **R** Raw

2 ripe avocados, peeled
¼ cup (60 mL) raw honey
¼ cup (60 mL) freshly squeezed lime juice
2 tbsp (30 mL) sweetened flaked or shredded coconut

Place all ingredients except coconut in a food processor or high-powered blender; process until nice and smooth. Give it a taste test, and if you prefer it sweeter, add more raw honey. Spoon into serving bowls and sprinkle with coconut.

. . . .

Joyous Tip

Want it a little sweeter but don't want to add honey?
Add 5 to 10 drops of liquid stevia, tasting after 5 drops
and adding more if you wish.

. . . .

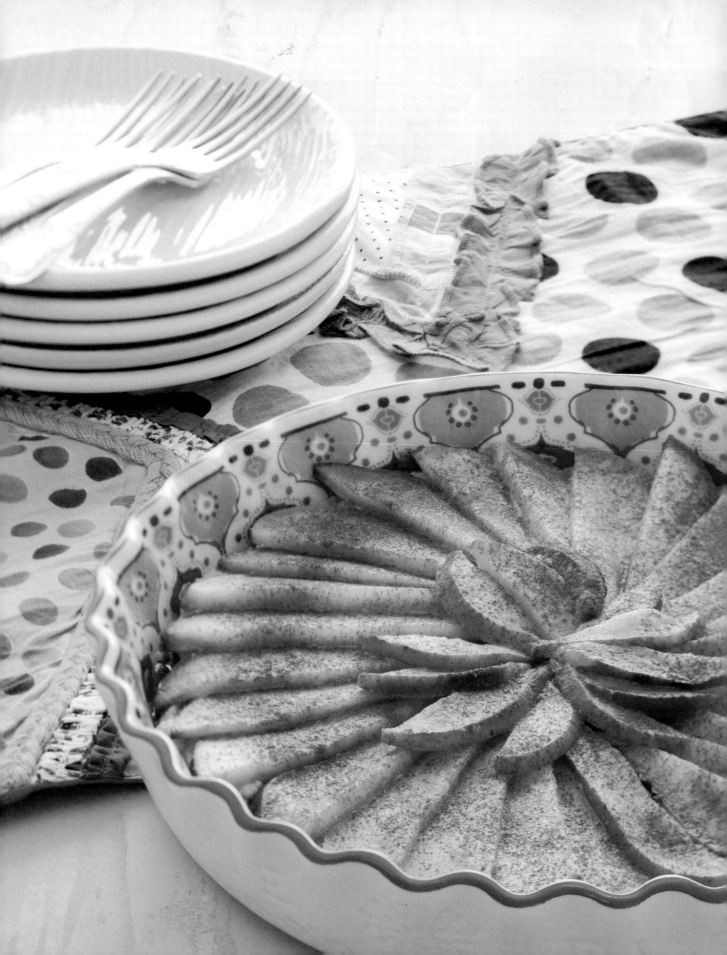

Pear Tart with Cashew Maple Cream

This is a summer potluck favorite of mine. Making it ahead and refrigerating it not only saves time but also makes for a fabulous chilled dessert. Or, in the winter, sauté the pears just before serving for a comforting Sunday-night dessert. Either way, remember to plan ahead: the cashews need to soak for 4 hours, and the dates for 1 hour.

Serves 8

Ⓥ Vegan   ⒹⒻ Dairy-free   ⒼⒻ Gluten-free   Ⓙ Joyous Comfort

Coconut Crust

1 cup (250 mL) pitted dates
  (soaked for 1 hour and
  drained well)

1½ cups (375 mL) walnuts
  or pecans

1 cup (250 mL) shredded
  or flaked coconut

Cashew Maple Cream

1 cup (250 mL) cashews
  (soaked for 4 hours and
  drained well)

3 tbsp (45 mL) coconut milk

2 tbsp (30 mL) real maple syrup

1 tsp (5 mL) pure vanilla extract

Pear Topping

2 tbsp (30 mL) coconut oil

3 large pears (unpeeled),
  washed, cored and
  thinly sliced

2 tsp (10 mL) cinnamon

2 tbsp (15 mL) real maple syrup

For the coconut crust, in a food processor, combine dates, walnuts and coconut; process until completely combined. Transfer mixture to a 9-inch (23 cm) pie plate; with moistened hands, firmly press crust into bottom and up sides of pan.

For the cashew maple cream, in a food processor or blender, combine cashews, coconut milk, maple syrup and vanilla; process until smooth like cream. Spread cashew cream in the crust. Cover and refrigerate for at least 2 hours before topping with pears.

For the pear topping, melt coconut oil in a large skillet over medium heat. Add pears and cook, gently stirring and turning, until soft, 10 to 15 minutes. Sprinkle with cinnamon and drizzle with maple syrup while cooking. Remove tart from the fridge and arrange sautéed pears on top of the cashew cream. Serve immediately or refrigerate overnight.

· ·

Joyous Tip

If you have a little cashew cream left over, serve each slice with a dollop on top. This recipe also works with any fruit, so use what's in season for the freshest and most nutrient-dense tart.

· ·

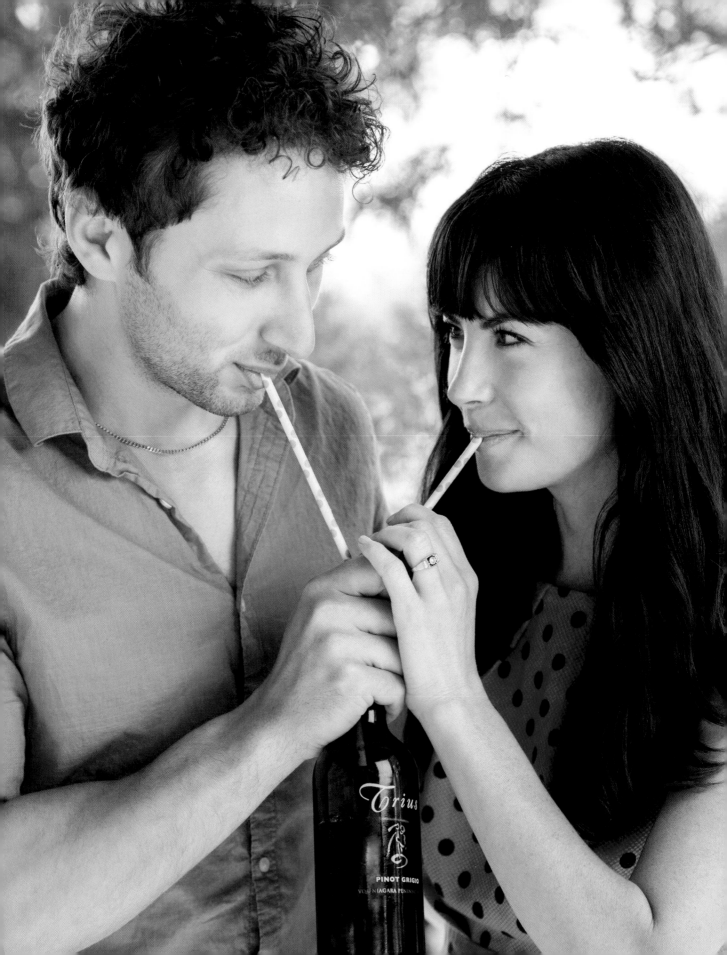

FINAL JOYOUS WORDS

Dear Joyous Health Reader,

Thank you for taking part in this joyous journey with me. I truly hope that what you've learned from my book inspires you to live a more joyous life! Remember that it's not just about what you eat, it's also about how you live your life, the thoughts you think and how often you move your sexy booty and get outside for fresh air. Reaching optimal health and preventing disease is a result of a holistic approach.

That being said, remember to avoid perfectionism and keep in mind that transitioning to joyous health takes time. Be kind to yourself and do not expect change overnight.

Lastly, I chose to share this photo of me and my sweet man, Walker, drinking local wine (from a polka-dot straw, of course!) because I want you to know that balance is very important. I drink wine, I eat chocolate—not every day, but I don't obsess about what I eat and drink. If I happen to be at an event or a family gathering where my usual healthy eats are not available, I don't have a meltdown or get stressed out that I'm going to fall off the wagon. If I happen to eat something not very joyous, I enjoy every bite of it, and I do not indulge in any food guilt whatsoever because I know I will be right back on track the next day. I recommend that you take the same approach! Or better yet, bring something joyous and healthy to that family gathering. Furthermore, when you make the change toward joyous health, you'll actually find it easy to stay on the path because you'll feel so much better.

FINAL JOYOUS THOUGHTS

When you focus on health and how you feel, as opposed to a number on the scale, you will find it far easier to reach your desired goals.

Every morsel you eat, every thought you think, is your choice! You have the power to make joyous choices to move you further toward incredible health and wellness.

Joyous Health to You!

Joy McCarthy, CNP, RNCP
Holistic Nutritionist, lover of real food

CONNECT WITH ME:
Blog: www.joyoushealth.ca—Join my Dose of Joy Newsletter
Twitter: @joyoushealth
Instagram: @joyoushealth
Facebook: facebook.com/joyoushealth.ca
Pinterest: joyoushealth

JOYOUS HEALTH FOOD AND WELLNESS JOURNAL

	BREAKFAST	LUNCH	DINNER	SNACKS	LIQUIDS
DAY 1					
	Time:	Time:	Time:	Time:	
	How are you feeling? Record your mood and any negative side effects of food.			BMs (bowel movements)	Exercise

	BREAKFAST	LUNCH	DINNER	SNACKS	LIQUIDS
DAY 2					
	Time:	Time:	Time:	Time:	
	How are you feeling? Record your mood and any negative side effects of food.			BMs (bowel movements)	Exercise

	BREAKFAST	LUNCH	DINNER	SNACKS	LIQUIDS
DAY 3					
	Time:	Time:	Time:	Time:	
	How are you feeling? Record your mood and any negative side effects of food.			BMs (bowel movements)	Exercise

	BREAKFAST	LUNCH	DINNER	SNACKS	LIQUIDS
DAY 4					
	Time:	Time:	Time:	Time:	
How are you feeling? Record your mood and any negative side effects of food.				BMs (bowel movements)	Exercise

	BREAKFAST	LUNCH	DINNER	SNACKS	LIQUIDS
DAY 5					
	Time:	Time:	Time:	Time:	
How are you feeling? Record your mood and any negative side effects of food.				BMs (bowel movements)	Exercise

	BREAKFAST	LUNCH	DINNER	SNACKS	LIQUIDS
DAY 6					
	Time:	Time:	Time:	Time:	
How are you feeling? Record your mood and any negative side effects of food.				BMs (bowel movements)	Exercise

	BREAKFAST	LUNCH	DINNER	SNACKS	LIQUIDS
DAY 7					
	Time:	Time:	Time:	Time:	
How are you feeling? Record your mood and any negative side effects of food.				BMs (bowel movements)	Exercise

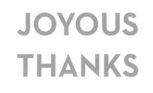

JOYOUS
THANKS

ACKNOWLEDGMENTS

After several years of working in marketing/advertising, I came to the realization that what I really wanted to do was to make a difference in people's lives in a more meaningful way than I was doing. So my first thank you is to the Institute of Holistic Nutrition, all the staff and all the teachers, especially Murat Vardar, whose encyclopedic knowledge of the human body ignited my passion and started me on my amazing joyous health journey.

Thank you to Walker Jordan, my love, my life partner, my best friend and official recipe taste tester—your unconditional love, humor and beautiful soul have inspired me to be the best version of myself. Of the seven billion people on planet Earth, you are one of a kind. I love you to infinity and beyond!

To Carol Dano, my creative guru who makes everything I do and think look joyous on the web or in print; to Kate McDonald Walker, my favorite nutrition nerd and wordsmith; and to Nicholas Collister, my photographer, who captured the essence of my joyous vision—thank you all from the bottom of my joyous heart!

Thank you to Andrea Magyar, my editor, and to Penguin Group (Canada) for believing in my joyous vision and bringing my dream to life with this, my first book. Thank you to my copy editor, Shaun Oakey, for his patience and eagle eye.

Thank you to all my clients worldwide and all the students I have had the opportunity to share my knowledge with. Your successes are my successes, and I am truly appreciative of each and every one of you.

So many individuals to mention, but a big thank you to all my family and friends … you know who you are! Your love and support have always inspired me to push myself to higher goals and aspirations.

Thank you to all my teachers over the years who taught me that it's not just what you eat but also the thoughts you think and how you treat your body that create a whole joyous healthy life.

Last but not least, a very joyous thanks to all my Joyous Health blog readers. You've inspired me to be the best I can possibly be in the kitchen and in life.

Cheers to joyous health!

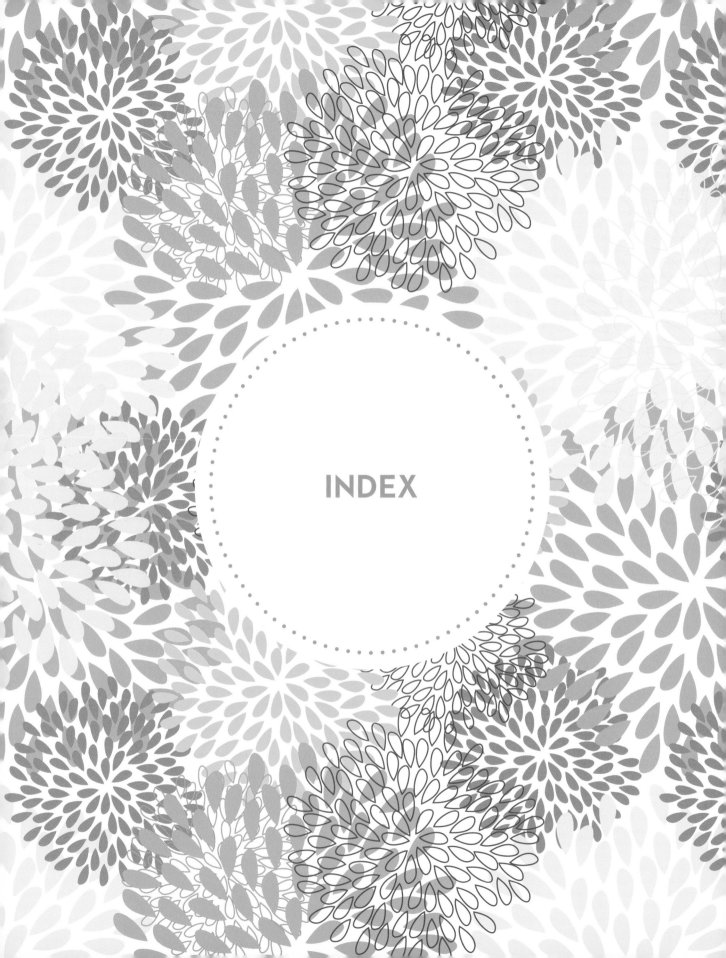

INDEX

A

alkalinizing
  juicing and, 172
  with lemon water, 12
allergies, 48
Allergies: Disease in Disguise
  (Bateson-Koch), 69
almond flour
  almond butter cookies, 219
  almond power muffins, 217
  apricot oat granola muffins, 139
goji berry muffins, 140
  rosemary crackers, 222
almonds
  power muffins, 217
  and vanilla milk, 170
almond sauce, 236
aloe vera juice, 39
American Chemical Society, 8
amino acids
  and digestion, 21
  and quinoa, 99
  role in digestion, 34
antacids, 25
antibiotics, natural, 95
anti-inflammatories
  in chicken soup, 179
  ginger, 95
  hemp seed, 96
  kale, 97
  quinoa, 99
antioxidants
  in coffee, 8
  in quinoa, 99
  in raw cacao, 100
  and superfoods, 88
apple cider vinegar, 28

apples
  beet and carrot slaw, 200
  cardamom crisp, 253
  and walnut French toast, 144
apricots: muffins, oat and
  granola, 139
artificial colors, 71–72
artificial flavors, 72
artificial sweeteners, 21
arugula
  and sun-dried tomato
    spelt pizza, 246
  and walnut pesto, 245
asparagus: roasted lemon
  with pecans, 241
avocado
  and cucumber soup, chilled, 182
  guac salsa, 233
  hemp seed guacamole, 210
  and kale tartine, 152
  matcha popsicles, 257

B

bacteria
  digestive, 32
  in large intestine, 23
  role of, 23, 31
baking powder, 123
baking soda
  test for stomach acid, 35
  types to purchase, 123
bananas
  and coconut flour pancakes, 148
  and maple grilled sandwich, 150
Bateson-Koch, Dr. Carolee, 69
bee pollen, 91
bee products as superfoods, 90–91

beet
  apple and carrot slaw, 200
  and goat cheese dip, 222
  soup, Thai, 189
beet test, 27
berries
  and blood sugar, 92
  blueberry spelt pancakes, 147
  and eye health, 92
  Morning Energizer blueberry
    smoothie, 165
  and quinoa, 142
  raspberry chocolate cheesecake
    smoothie, 162
  strawberry chia pudding, 157
  as superfoods, 92
betaine HCl
  and heartburn, 37
  test for stomach acid, 35
beverages. *See also* smoothies
  coconut milk, 168
  Detox Juice, 174
  Green Beauty Juice, 174
  Joyous Juices, 174
  limeade, 168
  sangria kombucha, 166
  Sunshine Juice, 174
bile, stimulation of, 12
bisphenol A (BPA), 75, 77
bitters, as digestive aid, 37
blender, 128

bloating
    calming tea for, 43
    and gum chewing, 21
    preventing, 38
blood sugar
    and chia seeds, 93
    effect of berries on, 92
    and insoluble fiber, 40
    and juice intake, 76
    and protein intake, 13, 14
    spirulina as stabilizer, 101
blueberries
    Morning Energizer
        smoothie, 165
    spelt pancakes, 147
body scan and mood, 56–57
bone health, 97
bowel movements. *See also*
    constipation
    apple cider vinegar as
        stimulant, 28
    beet test, 27
    and coffee, 9
    ideal, 26
    and lemon water, 12
BPA. *See* bisphenol A (BPA)
brain
    dump, and mood, 58
    fat in, 51
    role in eating, 20
bread
    almond flour rosemary
        crackers, 222
    bruschetta topping, 205
    French toast, with apples
        and walnut, 144

maple banana grilled
        sandwich, 150
    Mexican toast, 137
breads
    types to purchase, 118
    whole wheat and
        whole grain, 50
breakfast
    cereals, 78
    importance of, 13
    and insulin levels, 13
    recipes, 137–57
breast-feeding, advantages of, 33
broccoli: tamari, with
        sunflower seeds, 230
brownies: black bean chia, 267
bruschetta topping, 205
Brussels sprouts, spicy, 231
budget considerations, 125
burgers
    curry chicken, 227
    turkey, 233
butters: hemp seed
        maple cinnamon, 220

C

cacao, raw, 100
caffeine, 37. *See also* coffee
calcium, foods containing, 68
Candida, 31
carbohydrates
    for improved mood, 49
    order of eating, 36
    and snacks, 14
    source for good, 49

carrot(s)
    apple and beet slaw, 200
    cake balls, 258
    cake smoothie, 111
    and ginger soup, 180
cashew
    maple cream, 273
    millet mango salad, 198
    and orange cream, 254
cauliflower, mashed,
    with goat cheese, 244
cereals
    breakfast, 78
    types to purchase, 118
cheese, 122
chewing
    as gas and bloating
        preventative, 38
    importance of, 20
    and mindful eating, 7
    and saliva, 20
chia
    black bean brownies, 267
    and strawberry pudding, 157
chia seeds, 93
chicken
    curry, burgers, 227
    soup, Ma McCarthy's, 179
    stock, 182
chickpeas
    detox salad, 193
    sun-dried tomato hummus, 209
chicory, as alternative to coffee, 10
chili, tempeh, 239

chocolate
    and chili and cinnamon
        bark, 264
    gluten-free cookies, 262
    mint pudding, 270
    protein squares, 154
    and raspberry smoothie, 162
chyme, 21
coconut crust, 273
coconut flour
    almond power muffins, 217
    chocolate gluten-free
        cookies, 262
    pancakes with bananas, 148
coconut icing, 268
coconut milk, 168
coconut oil, 94
coffee
    advantages of, 8–9
    alternatives to, 10
    antioxidants in, 8
    and bowel movements, 9
    case history of decreasing
        intake, 11
    cutting back on, 9–10
    as diuretic, 8
    drawbacks to, 8, 9
    effect on body, 8
    limiting, and heartburn, 37
    and water consumption, 28
colon. *See* large intestine
condiments, 120

constipation. *See also* bowel
    movements
    case history, 24
    causes, 26, 29
    and coffee intake, 9
    and lemon water, 12
    probiotics as treatment, 31
    reducing, 27, 28–31, 30
    results of, 26
    and stress, 29
cookies
    almond butter, 219
    carrot cake balls, 258
    chocolate gluten-free, 262
    maca balls, 261
    trail mix, 263
corn syrup, high-fructose, 75
cosmetics, ingredients
    to avoid, 80
crackers: almond flour
    rosemary, 222
cucumber
    and avocado soup, chilled, 182
    tzatziki, 227

D

dairy
    alternatives to cow's milk, 123
    cheese, types to purchase, 122
    eliminating, and heartburn, 37
    products, as source of fat, 52
    yogurt, 75
David Suzuki Foundation, 81
Davis, Dr. William, 69

desserts
    recipes, 253–73
    when to eat, 36
detoxification
    foods for, 78
    foods to eliminate, 66–71
    and juicing, 172
    and lemon water, 12
    purpose, 66
    role of kale, 97
    of skin, 79
    smoothie for, 83
    of social circle, 82
    and spirulina, 101
Detox Juice, 174
detox salad dressing, 193
diarrhea, and stress, 29
diet
    food journal, 16
    increasing fiber in, 29
    wellness journal, 16
digestion, and kale, 97
digestive enzymes, 37
digestive system
    and amino acids, 21
    brain and, 20
    coffee as a stimulant to, 9
    effect of stress on, 29
    and gum chewing, 21
    and heartburn, 36–37
    and hydrochloric acid, 21
    liver and, 22
    mouth and, 20
    probiotics and, 31–33
    stomach and, 21

Digestive Wellness (Lipski), 31

Dijon honey salad dressing, 193

dips. *See also* spreads

    beet goat cheese, 222

    green pea and sun-dried

      tomato, 62

    tzatziki, 227

dry skin brushing, 79

E

Eat Well Feel Well, 59, 63

ecotherapy, 106

egg replacement, 122

eggs: avocado and kale tartine, 152

electric mixer, 129

Emmons, Dr. Robert, 110

emotional eating, 59–62

emotions, and disease, 58

Environmental Health

    Perspectives, 77

Environmental Working Group,

    75, 77, 80, 81, 104, 105

exercise

    benefits of, 37, 108

    and "forest bathing," 108

    and mood improvement, 57–58

eye health, and berries, 92

F

fats

    in chia seeds, 93

    in coconut oil, 94

    good, 51–52

    in hemp seeds, 96

    saturated and unsaturated, 52

    sources of good, 52

    types to purchase, 118

    in yogurt, 75

fiber

    benefits of, 40

    dietary, 40

    in fecal matter, 23

    foods rich in, 29, 42

    increasing in diet, 29

    and irritable bowel syndrome, 39

    role in digestion, 29

fish

    lemon pepper salmon, 228

    as source of fat, 52

flatulence, 38

flavonoids, 92

fluids. *See also* water

    drinking at meals, 36

folate, 53

food additives

    in cereals, 78

    colors, artificial, 71–72

    flavors, artificial, 72

    preservatives, artificial, 73

    sweeteners, artificial, 74

food diary, 61

food elimination

    and irritable bowel syndrome

      testing, 39

    and sensitivity testing, 30

food journal, 46

food labels, sugars listed on, 70

food poisoning, 22, 33

food processor, 129

Food Rules: An Eater's Manual

    (Pollan), 2

food(s). *See also* superfoods

    allergies, 48

    avoiding trigger, 59

    blue, 103

    bread: whole wheat

      and whole grain, 50

    breakfast cereals, 78

    budgeting for, 125

    canned, 75, 122

    color in, 103–4

    combining, and heartburn, 36

    containing fiber, 42

    elimination in detox diet, 66–71

    fats, 51–52

    fermented, types to

      purchase, 123

    fiber-rich, 29

    with good bacteria, 33

    green, 103

    health pyramid, 114–15

    and mood, 46–47, 49–53

    MSG in, 72

    nutrient rich, 29

    orange, 103

    packaged, avoiding, 2

recommended to avoid, 74–76
red, 103
to reduce constipation, 30
replacing with
    healthier, 126–27
seasonal, 125
sensitivities, 48
serving sizes, 118
spicy, and heartburn, 37
stocking pantry, 118–23
storage containers for, 130
water-dense, 29
yellow, 103
"forest bathing," 108
Forleo, Marie, 6
French toast, with apple and
    walnuts, 144
fruit
    combining with other foods, 36
    salad, 254
    sangria kombucha, 166
    types to purchase, 121
fruit juice, 76

G

gamma-linolenic acid, 96
gas
    preventing, 38
    production and gum chewing, 21
gazpacho, 184
ginger, 95
    and carrot soup, 180
    and lime vinaigrette, 198
gluten, eliminating, 37, 69
goat cheese
    and beet dip, 222
    and mashed cauliflower, 244

goji berry muffins, 140
granola: muffins, apricot
    and oats, 139
gratefulness, 110
Green Beauty Juice, 174
Green Goddess smoothie, 164
greens supplement, for irritable
    bowel syndrome, 39
guacomole, hemp seed, 210
gum chewing, 21, 38

H

headaches, 10
health food pyramid, 114–15
heartburn
    causes, 34
    reducing, 12, 36–37
heart disease
    and pumpkin seeds, 98
    and soluble fiber, 40
hemp
    milk, 170
    seed guacamole, 210
    seed maple cinnamon
        butter, 220
    seeds, 96
    and spinach pesto, 243
herbs, 97, 120
homogenization of milk, 66, 67
honey. *See also* bee products
    salad dressing, 200
    using, 91
hormones, 47–48
hugging, 109
hummus, sun-dried tomato, 209

hunger
    differentiated from thirst, 61
    reality check for, 60
hydrochloric acid
    and antacids, 25
    and digestive system, 21
    and food poisoning, 22

I

icing: coconut, 268
immune system
    foods to aid, 32
    ginger and, 95
In Defense of Food (Pollan), 74
insulin
    effect of snacks on, 14
    production and breakfast, 13
inulin, 241
irritable bowel syndrome, 39

J

Jensen, Dr. Bernard, 33
Joyous Juices, 174
juicer, 128
juices. *See* beverages
juicing, 172–73

K

kale, 97
    and avocado tartine, 152
    chips, cheesy, 208
    chips, curry-spiced, 206
    chips, lemon pumpkin seed sea
        salt, 206
    Green Goddess smoothie, 164
    orange and pecan salad, 202
    and walnut pesto, 245

kitchen makeover, 126–27

kitchen tools, 128–31

Knight, Stuart, 82

knives, 129

kombucha, sangria, 166

L

Lactobacillus acidophilus, 32

large intestine, 23–24

leaky gut syndrome, 23, 24

lemon

poppy seed loaf, 268

tahini drizzle for carrot ginger
soup, 180

lemon water, 28, 34, 36

benefits of, 12–13

and gas production, 38

lentil

curry loaf, 234

curry soup, 188

L-glutamine, 37

lifestyle, 106–10

Lijinsky, Dr. William, 73

limes

and ginger vinaigrette, 198

Key lime pudding, 271

limeade, 168

Lipski, Elizabeth, 31, 33

liver, 22

loaf, lemon poppy seed, 268

Logan, Dr. Alan, 106

Loving Body Scan, 56–57

M

magnesium, 98

mango

cashew and millet salad, 198

salsa, 227

margarine, 74

Mason jars, 130

meals

drinking liquids with, 36

size, and gas production, 38

10-day plan, 116–18

timing of, 36

metabolism: smoothie recipe
for boosting, 17

Mexican toast, 137

microwaved food, 74, 130

milk

alternative to cow's, 67, 123

coconut, 168

eliminating in detox diet, 66–68

goat's, 67

hemp, 170

vanilla almond, 170

millet, cashew and mango
salad, 198

mindful eating, 6–8, 20, 38

minerals, in superfoods, 89

mood

and fats, 53

and food relationship, 46–47

foods to improve, 49, 51, 52

and hormones, 47–48

improving, 49–53, 55–58

and nitric oxide, 47

and protein, 53

and trigger foods, 59

and vitamin D, 53

Morning Energizer blueberry
smoothie, 165

mouth, role in digesting, 20

MSG (monosodium
glutamate), 72

muffins

almond power, 217

apricot oat granola, 139

goji berry, 140

Murray, Dr. Michael, 39, 48

music, benefits of, 108

N

negative thoughts,
dispelling, 55–56

nitrates, 73

nitric oxide, and mood, 47

nitrites, 73

Northrup, Dr. Christiane, 47

nutrients

and detoxification, 172

foods rich in, 29

in hemp seeds, 96

and juicing, 172

in quinoa, 99

in raw cacao, 100

in smoothies, 161

nuts

and digestibility, 121

as source of fat, 52

types to purchase, 120

O

oats
  almond butter cookies, 219
  chocolate protein squares, 154
  muffins, apricot and
    granola, 139
oils
  as source of fat, 52
  stability and heat, 120
  types to purchase, 118
oranges
  and cashew cream, 254
  kale and pecan salad, 202

P

pancakes
  blueberry spelt, 147
  coconut flour banana, 148
parsnips, and pear soup, 186
pasta, 118
pasteurization, 66, 67
peaches and cream popsicles, 258
pears
  and parsnip soup, 186
  tart, 273
peas, green, and sun-dried
  tomato dip, 62
peppermint oil, for irritable
  bowel syndrome, 39
personal-care products
  coconut oil as, 94
  ingredients to avoid in, 80
  toxins in, 81
pesticides, avoiding, 104–5

pesto
  arugula walnut, 245
  hemp spinach, 243
  kale walnut, 245
  spinach walnut, 245
pies and tarts: pear tart, 273
pizza, sun-dried tomato arugula
  spelt, 246
Pollan, Michael, 2, 74
pop, 76
popcorn
  microwaved, 74
  turmeric sea salt, 212
popsicles
  avocado matcha, 257
  peaches and cream, 258
  raspberry maca, 257
potato salad, creamy herb, 197
preservatives, artificial
  effects of, 73
  in personal-care products, 80
probiotics
  and heartburn, 37
  role in digestion, 31–33
propolis, 91
protein
  animal, types to purchase, 121
  chia seeds as source, 93
  healthy options, 13
  hemp seeds as vegetarian
    source, 96
  and high-starch foods, 36
  importance of in diet, 13
  for improved mood, 50–51
  and insulin levels, 13

order of eating, 36
quinoa as source, 99
in smoothies, 161
in snacks, 14
sources, 51, 93, 96, 99
in spirulina, 101
vegetarian, types to
  purchase, 96, 122
pudding
  chocolate mint, 270
  Key lime, 271

Q

quinoa
  basic preparation, 137
  and berries, 142
  cardamom apple crisp, 253
  and grilled vegetable salad, 194

R

raspberry
  and chocolate cheesecake
    smoothie, 162
  maca popsicles, 257
royal jelly, 90–91

S

salads
  apple beet carrot slaw, 200
  chickpea detox, 193
  dressings,
    193, 194, 197, 198, 200, 202
  fruit, 254
  grilled vegetable quinoa, 194
  kale, orange, and pecan, 202
  mango cashew millet, 198
  potato, creamy herb, 197

saliva, and chewing, 20

salmon: lemon pepper, 228

salsa

guac, 233

mango, 227

sandwiches. *See also* wraps

avocado kale tartine, 152

maple banana grilled, 150

sangria kombucha, 166

sauces

almond, 236

arugula walnut pesto, 245

cashew orange cream, 254

hemp spinach pesto, 243

kale walnut pesto, 245

lemon pepper tahini, 228

spinach walnut pesto, 245

seaweeds, 121

seeds

chia, 93

as source of fat, 52

types to purchase, 121

Selhub, Dr. Eva, 106

sensitivities, food, 48

serving sizes, 118

skin

care, and pumpkin seeds, 98

detoxifying, 79

improving with lemon water

drink, 12

sleep

benefits of, 37, 109–10

and emotional eating, 62

and irritable bowel

syndrome, 39

small intestine, function of, 23

smoothies

carrot cake, 111

Clean Beauty, 83

Green Goddess, 164

metabolism booster for

breakfast, 17

Morning Energizer, 165

protein in, 161

raspberry chocolate

cheesecake, 162

superfoods in, 161

snacks

and emotional eating, 62

high in sugar, 14

and insulin levels, 14

protein in, 14

recipes, 206–22

suggestions for healthy, 14

superfood trail mix, 215

turmeric sea salt popcorn, 212

soft drinks, 76

soup

cardamom parsnip pear, 186

carrot ginger, 180

chicken, 179

chicken stock, 182

cucumber and avocado,

chilled, 182

curry lentil, 188

gazpacho, 184

Thai beet, 189

turkey stock, 182

soy, eliminating in detox

diet, 70–71

spelt flour

lemon poppy seed loaf, 268

pancakes, with blueberries, 147

sun-dried tomato arugula

pizza, 246

trail mix cookies, 263

spices, 97, 120

spinach

Green Goddess smoothie, 164

and hemp pesto, 243

and walnut pesto, 245

spirulina, 101

spreads. *See also* dips

bruschetta topping, 205

hemp seed guacamole, 210

hemp seed maple cinnamon

butter, 220

sun-dried tomato hummus, 209

tzatziki, 227

squares

black bean chia brownies, 267

chocolate protein, 154

squash, spaghetti, with

chia seeds, 248

stock: chicken and turkey, 182

stomach

acid in, 21, 34

role in digestion, 21

tests for acid in, 35

storage containers, 130

strawberry chia pudding, 157

stress
and diarrhea, 29
effect on digestion, 29
and emotional eating, 59–60
and gas production, 38
and irritable bowel
syndrome, 39
reduction, and heartburn, 37
sugar
eliminating in detox diet, 70
identifying on labels list, 70
and irritable bowel
syndrome, 39
spikes caused by coffee, 8
types to purchase, 123
Sunshine Juice, 174
superfoods
additions to top 12, 104
antioxidants in, 88
bee products, 90–91
benefits of, 86–87
berries, 92
chia seeds, 93
coconut oil, 94
ginger, 95
hemp seeds, 96
herbs, 97
kale, 97
minerals in, 89
pumpkin seeds, 98
quinoa, 99
raw cacao, 100
and smoothies, 161
spices, 97
spirulina, 101

squash seeds, 98
top 12, 90
types to purchase, 123
vitamins in, 89
superfood trail mix, 215
supplements
to aid digestion, 37
for irritable bowel
syndrome, 39
probiotic, 31–33
sweeteners, artificial, 74
sweets, 122

T

tea: anti-bloat stomach-
calming, 43
teas
black, caution about, 9
recommended, 37
types to purchase, 120
teeccino (coffee alternative), 10
tempeh chili, 239
10-day meal plan, 116–18
*Thanks! How the New Science
of Gratitude Can Make You
Happier* (Emmons), 110

tomatoes
bruschetta topping, 205
gazpacho, 184
sun-dried, and green pea dip, 62
sun-dried, arugula spelt
pizza, 246
tools, kitchen, 128–31
traditional Chinese medicine:
perspective on liver, 22
trail mix
cookies, 263
superfood, 215
trigger foods, 59
turkey
burgers, 233
stock, 182
type 2 diabetes
and high-sugar snacks, 14
and insoluble fiber, 40
tzatziki, 227

U

Ulrich, Robert, 106
urine, color as gauge of
hydration, 28
Uy, Michelle, 59, 63

V

vegetables
  nutrients in, 13
  types to purchase, 121
  vitamins in, 172
vegetables, grilled,
  and quinoa salad, 194
vinaigrette: lime ginger, 198
vinegar: cider and bowels, 28
vitamin B_6, 72
vitamin B_{12}, 53
vitamin D, 53
vitamin E, 98
"vitamin G," 106
vitamins
  in kale, 97
  in spirulina, 101
  in superfoods, 89
  in vegetables, 172

W

walking, as mood improver, 58
water
  as aid to liver function, 22
  calculating daily
    requirements, 115
  and coffee consumption, 28
  and lemon drink, 12–13, 28
  and mealtimes, 61
  as morning drink, 8
  to reduce constipation, 28
  types to purchase, 123
weight control, and coconut oil, 94
wellness journal, 16, 276–77
wheat, eliminating in detox
  diet, 69
Wheat Belly (Davis), 69
Women's Bodies, Women's Wisdom
  (Northrup), 47
wraps: Raw Sunshine, 236

Y

yogurt, 75
  tzatziki, 227
Your Brain on Nature
  (Selhub and Logan), 106, 108

Z

zinc, 98
zucchini pasta, 243

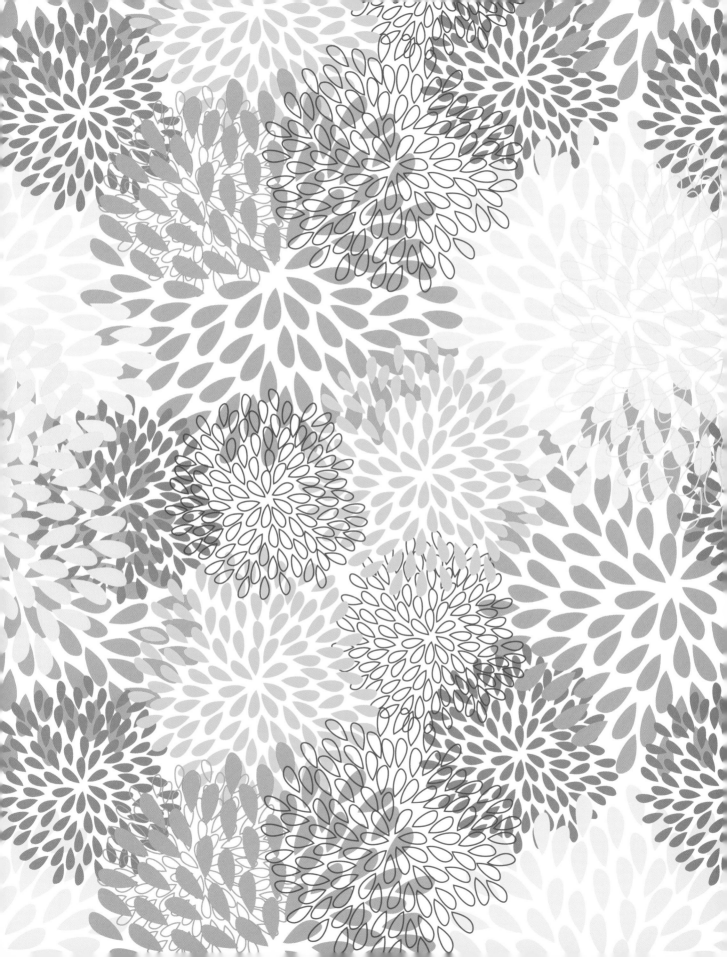

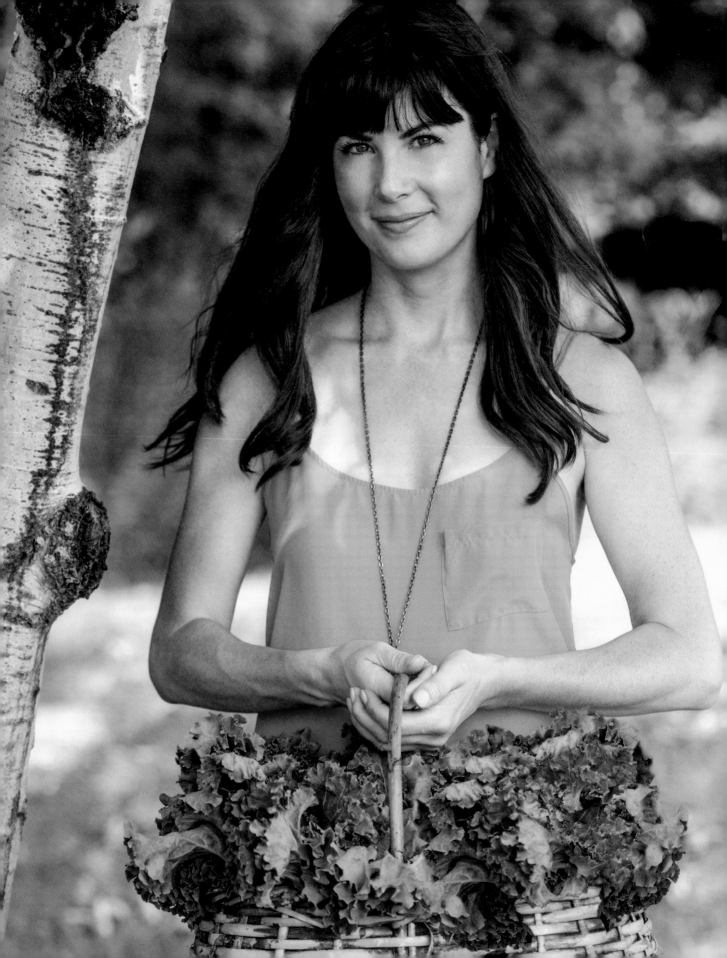